CRUISE SHIP OR NURSING HOME

THE 5 ESSENTIALS OF A MAXIMIZED LIFE

LERNER | LOMAN | MAJORS | PELLOW | SHUEMAKE

Maximized Living™
1170 Celebration Blvd., Suite 100B, Celebration, FL 34747

Published in Orlando, Florida, by Maximized Living™ Publishing, Inc.

In view of the complex, individual nature of health and fitness problems, this book, and the ideas, programs, procedures, and suggestions are not intended to replace the advice of trained medical professionals. All matters regarding one's health require medical supervision. A physician should be consulted prior to adopting any program or programs described in this book, or any of the Maximized Living™ resources. The contents of this book are based upon the opinions of the authors. The authors and publisher disclaim any liability arising directly or indirectly from the use of this book.

This book is not intended to make recommendations related to getting on or off prescription or over-the-counter medication. If you face any current health concerns, or are currently taking medication, it is always recommended to seek the advice of your physician before starting a new nutrition or fitness program. While many of the testimonials shared in this book show patients getting well and then getting off of their medications, only your medical doctor can prescribe drugs or tell you to get off of drugs. Our role is to make you aware of the hazards of poor lifestyle decisions while helping you to create optimum function and healing in your body. In time, you must begin to judge for yourself whether your medications are keeping you alive, merely palliating symptoms of an unhealthy body, or actually causing some of the ailments you suffer from. With the guidance of your prescribing physician, you need to make your own best decisions on medication. As you heal, work with your medical doctors to help you reduce or eliminate the drugs you're on.

The information in this book is intended to be education and should not replace consultation with a competent healthcare professional. The content of Cruise Ship or Nursing Home is intended to be used as an adjunct to responsible healthcare supervised by a healthcare professional. The authors and Maximized Living™ are not liable for any misuse of the material contained in this book.

ISBN10:193393699-1
ISBN13: 9781933-936994

Library of Congress Cataloging-in-Publication Data

Lerner, Ben; Loman, Greg; Majors, Charles; Pellow, Chris; Shuemake, Eric
    Cruise Ship or Nursing Home
        p. cm.
    ISBN10:193393699-1
    ISBN13: 9781933-936994
    1. Health   2. Nutrition   3. Happiness
        I. Ben Lerner.   II. Title

For more information about Maximized Living™ or to obtain additional copies of *Cruise Ship or Nursing Home*, please contact Maximized Living™ at 321-939-3060 or info@MaximizedLiving.com.

Printed in the United States of America

C O N T E N T S

INTRODUCTION

What This Book Is and What
This Program Can Do for You

*"We have so much time,and so little to do!
Strike that; reverse it."[1]*

—*Gene Wilder as Willy Wonka*

This Book Is Not Complicated

If you are looking for the next biggest secret to the fountain of youth, we have news for you; it doesn't exist. The answer to your health problems isn't the latest ab toner, thigh blaster, or some mystical berry from the Amazon jungle.

While the science we will share with you is cutting edge, the answers are simple. What we have discovered is that the most life-changing truths are easy—not hard—to follow. If you cooperate with the way your body was designed to work, you get health and look and feel your best. If you don't cooperate, you get disaster—period. The problem is that most people don't know how they were designed. This book will change that. You will learn from many people how simple it is to radically transform your health, lose hundreds of pounds, get off countless medications, restore your energy, and reverse the affects of numerous diseases. The best part? It's not complicated.

This Program Has Worked Over and
Over and Over Again. It Does Not Fail

It may be simple, but you still have to do it! The reason everything from home exercise equipment and diet books to drugs, surgery, and our entire health care system has totally failed is because you have to change in order for your health and body to change. If information, equipment, and pills changed lives, you'd already be changed. Only action changes people. Nothing else does. Part 2 of this book is your action plan. We have laid out a 28 day challenge that will give you the day by day eating plan with recipes, specific exercise program to maximize your hormone response, detox system and most of all, the tools to change your mindset so that these changes actually stick.

> Only action changes people. Nothing else does.

This isn't a 28 day diet. Diets don't work. It is your entrance ramp to a new way of viewing and managing your health. One that has worked with thousands of patients that you will meet in this book. It is not unusual to see people lose 10-15 pounds in two weeks, normalize their blood pressure in three weeks and actually start developing a six pack of abs in four weeks. If you want to skip ahead to the action plan, go for it!

This Book Offers Hope

Lasting change is 80 percent behavior and 20 percent education. This book will give you the steps to take immediate action, but most importantly it will give you hope—the hope that you can overcome whatever hand you have been dealt or whatever diagnosis you've been given. This book will help you develop healthy habits and change your behavior forever!

This Book Is Written by Doctors Who Still See Results with Real Patients Every Day

We have combined over 50 years of clinical experience dealing with literally tens of thousands of patients with thousands of different medical conditions and ailments. You've seen hundreds of books about health and fitness. Chances are you have at least five on your shelves right now. The problem is they don't work. That's why we call them "shelf-help" books. These books are selling millions, but the reason they're helping almost no one is that what's written in them has never been tested or proven to be reproducible. Our offices, however, have been our "living laboratories." What we teach has been tried and proven in our offices and in hundreds of offices around the world. We only write about the real-life results we're seeing every day.

We Practice What We Preach

We also practice what we preach in our own families. We wouldn't show you this program if we couldn't keep it up consistently at home. **The bottom line:** this stuff works!

This Program Is Not Like Every Other Health Program Out There

In recent years, diet books have ruled the top of the best-sellers lists, and you can sign up for dozens of weight-loss programs in clinics, gyms, doctor offices, and online. All promise quick, permanent weight loss and the well-being of your dreams. Despite all of the promises, obesity has skyrocketed. Worst of all, childhood obesity has gone into hyperspace for kids. Nine million kids under the age of six are now obese! Over two million people are dying unnecessarily every year from cancer and heart disease. We're more depressed than ever, and the flu scare is worse every year. The current ideas and programs on health and fitness clearly aren't working. How is it working for you? It's not, so stop listening to the ads and quit following the fads. We will help you understand the true scientific reasons for lasting weight loss, time saving exercise, true detox, and how together, these truly lead to what you're looking for. You don't need another colon cleanse or fad diet. You need to learn the real steps to show you how to make a permanent, not just day or weeklong changes. If you want to fit into your skinny clothes again, or just feel better, you will learn things in this book that you have never heard before. It's about time!

> You don't need another colon cleanse or fad diet. You need to learn the real steps to show you how to make permanent, not just day or weeklong, changes.

How Is this Maximized Living Book Different?

Instead of a "how to" book, this is a "how to do it" book. We will show you how to take five simple steps toward the life and health of your dreams, and you will meet people who are just like you and had the same conditions you have. You will learn how they gained victory over their diagnoses and took control of their futures.

We're going to coach you step-by-step through the makeover you will experience as we journey together down the road of Maximized Living. In fact, we look forward to the time when you send in your story so we can see, and hopefully share with the world, how your life has been transformed.

Our Promise

Our promise to you is this: if you follow the guidelines of this proven system, your health will never be the same again. Your friends will be looking at you and wondering what the heck happened. You will be an amazing role model for your family, who ultimately follow your actions and not your words. You will leave them with a health legacy that will be passed on from generation to generation. Your grandchildren and great-grandchildren will personally be indebted to you for your efforts. And perhaps most importantly; they'll be partying with you on a cruise ship and not visiting you in a nursing home.

CHAPTER 1

Cruise Ship or Nursing Home?
Your Road Map to a Maximized Life

"You're looking at a man who is not walking through the valley of the shadow of death. He's galloping into it!"[1]

—*Anthony Hopkins as William Parrish in Meet Joe Black*

The Most Important Health Question You Will Ever Answer

WHERE DO YOU WANT TO BE when you are sixty or seventy? On a cruise ship, staring at the sun setting over the ocean, or stuck in a nursing home, staring at a bucket of pills?

When you reach a fork in the road, you have to pick one or the other—and you, my friend, are at that fork, whether you know it or not. By not choosing the path you will walk down today, you are choosing the nursing home path by default. The simple fact is this; if you are anything like the thousands of patients we see every day in our offices and if you continue what you are doing now, the odds are stacked against you ever making it to that cruise ship. The path that almost everyone around you is on is the path to the nursing home. Many of them (and possibly you) are not walking down that path but sprinting down it. Think about it. If you take a thousand people in this country, where do 999 of them end up? That's right, in the nursing home, dependent on others, or worse—dying tragically early.

Now here's the problem: if we asked all of those same people when they were twenty-five, thirty, forty, or fifty years old where they thought they were going to end up, what do you think they would have said? They would've said, "On the cruise ship!"

You see, nobody intends to end up in the nursing home, but your intentions don't determine where you will end up, your actions do. This program is meant to change your actions. Changing your actions will also change your path and give you one with a future. Tens of thousands of people have taken the steps toward the cruise ship by taking the simple steps in this book. If you are ready to get on the fast track to a great life and an incredible future, this book is your road map. By the time you finish the five simple steps, you will be galloping down the path to the cruise ship.

THE FIVE ESSENTIALS:
What Are They and Why Do They Matter to Me?

"This will bring health to your body and nourishment to your bones."
—*Proverbs* 3:8, *NIV*

Your body needs no help to heal you; it just needs no interference. If you get this one principle, it will change your life and your health forever.

Read that statement again. Now let it sink in for a minute. Your body is an incredible self-healing machine. You are not defective or helpless. At your core, you lack nothing to be healthy—not a pill, a shot, or anything else. If you nick yourself shaving today, what would happen in a couple of days? It would heal. Healing is in the package. It's free, and there are no side effects. There is no doctor or drug on the planet that can heal that cut for you. Only your body can do it. So if your body can heal a cut on your leg or face today, why is it that you are reading this with high blood pressure, acid reflux, sleep problems, diabetes, or headaches? Why isn't your body healing those things? It's because something is interfering with that healing power.

> Your body is an incredible self-healing machine. You are not defective or helpless.

If you find the source of the interference, you find the cause of your problem. If you remove the cause of the problem, your body can heal. We've seen people heal of all of the above conditions by removing the interference. Just give your body what it needs and you will be amazed at what it can do, no matter how bad you think things have gotten.

What may really shock you is that something is also interfering with your "leaning" power—the body's inherent ability to get and stay lean. That's right, you were designed to be lean—like those people you hate who eat what they want and still look ripped. You've just interfered. Interference, however, can be avoided or removed.

That's Where the Five Essentials Come In

There are Five Essentials to Maximized Living, and we call them "Essentials" because each one is absolutely necessary to live the full, abundant life you were intended to live. Do any less and you suffer the consequences. These Five Essentials are irreducible minimums to keep the cells in your body regenerating instead of degenerating, and fit instead of fat.

A lot of health experts attempt to dilute health down to only one discipline or essential. For example, they might say, "It's all about nutrition." Nothing, however, could be further from the truth. Yes, it is important to eat well, but if you ignore the other four components of Maximized Living, your body will not even be able to digest the good food you have eaten. Yes, it is wonderful to work out and have muscles, but if you ignore the other essentials, you may end up a miserable, albeit muscular, person who will look great in a coffin someday. Jim Fixx, the creator of jogging, died of a heart attack—while jogging. Clearly something is missing in today's world of "wellness."

> These Five Essentials are irreducible minimums to keep the cells in your body regenerating instead of degenerating, and fit instead of fat.

Our only goal in this book is to help you reach your potential, which is greater than you can probably imagine at this point. Your body is like a Ferrari, but you've never gotten out of second gear. It's time to take off the limits! To reach your true health potential and to lead a long, joyful, and fulfilling life, you have to address all of the Five Essentials. It's not about perfecting all five, because health food nuts, superior athletes, and stress gurus don't necessarily live better, longer lives. It's about consciously paying attention to and intentionally living by the principles of the Five Essentials. By applying these principles, you give yourself the best chance of getting what you really, truly want—a maximized life!

What Are the Five Essentials?

After years of research, study, and treating people of all ages, shapes, and sizes, the Five Essentials we have discovered are:

ESSENTIAL No. 1: Maximized Mind
ESSENTIAL No. 2: Maximized Nerve Supply
ESSENTIAL No. 3: Maximized Quality Nutrition
ESSENTIAL No. 4: Maximized Oxygen and Lean Muscle
ESSENTIAL No. 5: Minimized Toxins

While most of these may seem commonsensical at first glance, it is amazing how many of us do not practice any—let alone all—of the Five Essentials on a regular, daily basis. You say you want to eat well, but do you understand what that really means? Do you know what the "good" foods really are? You may take deep breaths and exercise when you can, but do you know the best ways to get oxygen deep into your tissues and the right ways to build muscles so that they keep your body running at its peak? If you answer honestly, most people don't—and if you don't know how to live those two essentials, chances are good that you don't fully understand how the other three can help or hurt you either.

Let's take a look at why the Five Essentials are so crucial to your overall well-being and how they work with each other to produce Maximized Lives.

How Do the Essentials Work?

It's a question every good mother asks, "Are you taking care of yourself?" It's even a substitute for good-bye: "Hey, take care of yourself," or "Take care!"

Here's a really big question: What does it mean to "take care of yourself"? Remember, your body needs no help. Just remove the interference so that it can heal and be lean. Therefore, taking care of yourself equals removing components of your lifestyle that are out of alignment with how your body was designed to work.

Taking care of yourself goes hand in hand with the Five Essentials. These essentials are like gravity. Gravity is a law. You don't have to like it or even know about it, but it will impose itself on you every single time. You can choose to live your life in accordance with the Five Essentials or not, but they will not be ignored.

There is only one way to well-being. It's not treatment; it's care. Any doctors, treatments, or recommendations that don't line up with the Five Essentials will not ultimately hold up or create results. This is why we're currently in the shape we're in—out of shape. Caring for the body by removing interference and ultimately living a life that creates little interference in the first place is real health care. It's the law, and the only real way to long-term well-being.

As you take the five steps away from the nursing home and toward the cruise ship, you will be applying the Five Essentials of Maximized Living.

Testimonial — *Hank Henningsen and family*

The Five Essential Keys to Happiness

I am here to tell you there really is hope out there. I am living proof. Maximized Living pulled me out of a deep pit of depression. They saved my life, my job, and my family.

I can't begin to tell you how miserable my life had become. It seems so far away now. Back then, I suffered (and I mean suffered) from severe depression, serious weight problems (298 pounds), anxiety, insomnia, and sleep apnea. I spent three hundred dollars a month on medications and at least another three hundred dollars per month on psychotherapy and twelve-step programs.

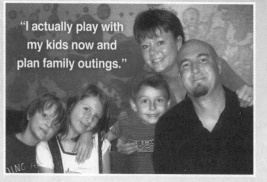

"I actually play with my kids now and plan family outings."

But worst of all, I always wanted to be alone. Any kind of social interaction made me want to crawl into a hole. As outlets for my anxiety, I developed dangerous addictions, primarily to tobacco and alcohol. All of this made me truly hate myself. I felt so worthless that I could barely look my wife and kids in the face, so I didn't spend any time with them. You can imagine how rejected that made them feel. We were falling apart as a family. On top of that, I was losing my job. I was only thirty-five.

Maximized Living rescued me. After attending some seminars, I learned about the Five Essentials and decided that it was time to make a change. My family was worth it! I went on the Advanced Eating Plan for two weeks, then I did a cellular cleansing for two weeks. Pretty soon I had switched to grass-fed, not grain-fed, beef. I started eating breakfast and lunch instead of just dinner and stopped putting sugar in my coffee. We banned sodas from our house and installed a water filtration system instead. I threw out our non-organic cleaners and replaced all of our plastic containers with glass. I wanted to make our lives over completely.

The result of all this? I lost 40 pounds in 90 days and another 30 in the next six months. That really lifted my mood. Soon I was able to break off my alcohol and tobacco addictions entirely. I even stopped all the mood and pain medications. I don't need them anymore. That is a miracle to me. I am depression-free!

As I lost all the old bad habits, I gained hope and happiness. I actually play with my kids now and plan family outings. I haven't used my sleep apnea machine in months. My concentration has improved dramatically and the social anxiety is much better. The funny thing is, I actually eat more now than I did when I weighed almost 300 pounds. The difference is that now I eat well without gaining weight. Soon I will start surge training with the goal of losing another 30 pounds. I totally believe I will succeed. Life looks good to me now!

But that's not all. My family follows the Five Essentials and we are healthier than I ever thought we could be. Our lives are 100 percent different than they were a year ago and 100 percent better. That's why I say Maximized Living saved my life.

Example of the Five Essentials at Work

Here's how interfering with or ignoring the Five Essentials plays a major role in developing depression (or any illness):

Interfering with or Ignoring Essential 1:
The unmaximized mind

Lack of sleep, poor self-image, and too much stress are at an all-time high right now. They all cause neurotransmitter burnout, increased stress hormones, chronic fatigue, and destructive, self-loathing thoughts. Resolving these problems through Essential 1 is the first step to overcoming depression.

Interfering with or Ignoring Essential 2:
Damage or misalignment of the spine and nervous system

Vertebral misalignment and poor posture create tension and interference within the central nervous system. The nervous system is responsible for controlling gland function, and glands control the balance of body chemistry. You will meet many people in this book who have overcome depression, largely due to spinal correction, through adherence to Essential 2.

Interfering with or Ignoring Essential 3:
Poor nutrition

Diets high in carbohydrates leave a constant level of insulin in the system, which lowers Serotonin levels and causes inflammation. Imbalances in Omega-3 and Omega-6 ratios have been found to be the first factor to address regarding depression, according to professors at Harvard and Oxford universities. Stimulants, sugars, and artificial additives negatively affect blood sugar levels and alter brain function. Nutrient deficiency can be solved by food and supplementation, which is the key part of Essential 3.

Interfering with or Ignoring Essential 4:
Sedentary lifestyle

Inactivity and a lack of intentional exercise has many damaging effects upon function and mental health. That's why, in medical studies, exercise consistently matches or exceeds the benefits of antidepressants.

Interfering with or Ignoring Essential 5:
High levels of toxicity

Toxins and chemicals found, for example, in medications and refined foods, affect hormone balance and glandular function.

Listed above are just a few crucial factors related to the Five Essentials and depression. Think about it: you can walk through virtually every condition related to health and fitness today and discover it's connection to the Five Essentials. Thousands of studies support this law. We will show you how to easily incorporate the Five Essentials of Maximized Living to guarantee you are in fact "taking care of yourself."

CHAPTER 2

You've Been Lied To!

*"I never could tell a lie that anybody would doubt
nor a truth that anybody would believe."*[1]

—*Mark Twain*

AT OUR SEMINARS, WE ACTUALLY have people stand up, point at the people around them and yell, "You've been lied to!" You should look in the mirror and say it to yourself, because what you have been taught about your health is a big fat hairy lie—a lie that is keeping you in bondage to the drug companies, your sickness, and/or a body you don't want. What's worse is that what you believe to be true isn't true! At the beginning of each action step and throughout the book, you will discover the lies that have been holding you back and the actual truths that will set you free.

Here's the first one:

YOU'VE BEEN LIED TO!

LIE: It's not going to happen to me.

TRUTH: It's already happening to you.

As doctors that have worked with hundreds of thousands of patients, let us assure you of something: denial is a terrible strategy for your health. It doesn't work because the reality always catches up to you. There are two things that you can do with truth:

1. You can let it transform you.
2. You can deny its existence and let it ruin you.

In the end, there is no escaping the truth.

Another bad strategy is procrastination. When it comes to your body and your life, "tomorrow" is often too late. You need a new strategy—a strategy that doesn't start with, "It's not going to happen to me." Frankly, that strategy will kill you.

The simple truth is that you cannot wait for a diagnosis or a crisis to make a change in your health. That's too late. By that time, you are fighting a battle that you usually don't win. Diabetes, heart disease, cancer, Alzheimer's, and almost every other disease that will rob you of your future have one thing in common: they form in your body long before you detect them. Unless you're consciously doing something to prevent them, one of those deadly diseases is destroying your body as you sit here reading this book.

> You cannot wait for a diagnosis or a crisis to make a change in your health. That's too late. By that time, you are fighting a battle that you usually don't win.

Disease occurs now. It just kills you later. What you do today, how your body is functioning, what drugs you're on, and how well you take care of yourself determine your future. Most people live today like there is no tomorrow and for many Americans, there isn't.

The worst part about diseases is not death; it's the suffering, misery, and loss of potential. The worst part about diabetes isn't dying; it's sitting in a dialysis center three days a week for five hours a day and not being able to work or support your family. It's having your toes or other body parts amputated because they ache to the bone and have oozing sores that you can't stand anymore. The worst part about having a stroke isn't leaving your kids or grandkids behind when you die. It's having them take care of you or visit you in a nursing home where others are taking care of you—while you are still alive for ten more excruciating years.

Sound scary? At least it's the truth and not a lie. Change your strategy. Don't wait for these end-stage events to happen. Take control now like it will happen to you if you don't.

Patient Story

In our offices, we meet couples every day like Ron and Marilyn. Again, if you do what everyone else does, you will have what everyone else has. **This is a true story.**

Ron and Marilyn never really took care of their health. Neither of them had ever exercised on a consistent basis, and their nutritional habits were less than desired. Robert had been a smoker most of his life and tried to stop without much luck. Neither of them invested in their health. Then the moment came when they wished they had.

Two days before their 21 wedding anniversary, Ron's left hand felt heavy. He went to pick up his fork but noticed he couldn't. Could he be having a stroke? By the time he was rushed to the emergency room, his entire left side was paralyzed. The next five days, as Ron described them, "were the worst days of my life."

> Unless you're Bill Gates, you're just one serious illness away from bankruptcy.

The neurologist said there was nothing medical science could do for him since the culprit blood vessel was too deep in his brain. Ron was sent home never to be able to work or function at 100 percent again.

Marilyn had never worked. She was a stay-at-home mom. Ron's medical expenses were staggering and their health insurance policy only paid a portion. Within three years they had spent over $300,000 out of pocket on medical bills. Their nest egg was down to nothing, and they were at risk of losing their home. An attorney specializing in medical bankruptcy even suggested they look at getting a divorce and making Marilyn liable for the remaining medical bills, so that she could file bankruptcy and have all the bills expunged.

Dr. David Himmelstein, an associate professor of medicine at Harvard University, commented: "Unless you're Bill Gates, you're just one serious illness away from bankruptcy. Most of the medical bankruptcies were average Americans who happened to get sick."[2] Many people think that insurance will protect them, but tragically 75 percent of people who filed for bankruptcy also had health insurance.[3]

After entering one of our offices, Ron was asked, "If you could say one thing to people, what would you say?" He sighed, "Invest in your health while you have the chance."

Dr. Pellow's Story

By Dr. Chris Pellow

At some point in my late twenties, the poor attention I was giving to my life had me in debt up to my eyeballs, and the poor attention I was giving to my body left me at 250 pounds and completely out of shape. I was mostly angry and saddened at how I felt about myself. On the outside I told myself everything was fine and I should just put on a happy face, but on the inside I just knew I wasn't being honest.

Thankfully, I came upon a morning that changed my life forever. I was at a seminar where there was a morning jog on the schedule, and I decided to participate. On that jog, I came face-to-face with the realization of how bad I had gotten. I watched as all of my friends repeatedly lapped me. I had been in total denial for years. This wake-up call was more painful and annoying than the hotel wake-up call at 5:00 a.m. When I got back to the room after the run (OK, walk), the person that looked back at me in that hotel mirror didn't look happy at all. I finally accepted the truth: I needed to change and I needed to change now!

I came to a place that morning where I realized that if I could manage the person in the mirror, I could win and live the life of my dreams. I decided to transform my life and start doing the steps in this book. Since then, I have completed a marathon in 4.5 hours and climbed mountains. My renewed body and my new life have led me to help thousands of patients and others just like you. Your first step on Day 1 of the challenge is to get real with yourself. You may have lived with your health problems for so long that they seem like part of your normal life. It's time to look at where you are, what your risk factors are and why you want to do something about it. Go to the "Man or woman in the mirror" section of day 1 in the challenge and complete the exercise there.

You Are Not a Victim

The road to Maximized Living begins with a challenge. For better or for worse, you are the ruler of your future. The challenge is for you to change. Changing homes, spouses, diet books, gyms, churches, cities, or doctors won't make the difference. To experience change, you need to change. There's a great old saying, "Wherever you go, there you are."

The Maximized Living challenge to get you moving away from the nursing home and toward the cruise ship isn't theory. It works every single time, and it starts with acknowledging that you are responsible for your health and your future. Your situation isn't your spouse's fault. It isn't your parents' fault. It isn't your friends' or co-workers' faults. It's yours. You can continue to blame your circumstances or those around you for your problems, but how's that working out for you?

> To experience change, you need to change.

The fact that it's your fault is good news, because you can't always change others or the things around you, but, believe it or not, you can always change you. You are not dependant on anyone or anything else. We see lives turn around in a hurry when people accept that fact. So accept responsibility, and let's get to work!

To get on the path toward the cruise ship and away from the nursing home, you need to take only five steps. These five steps will incorporate all of the Five Essentials of Maximized Living. It's simple, easy, and works every time. The journey of a thousand miles begins with a single step, and taking the steps is all we're asking you to do.

Testimonial *– Kaila Beattie, 32 years old*

100 Pounds and Still Going Strong

For any mother reading this, you might understand the feeling of gaining the extra forty to fifty pounds with pregnancy, then working hard to lose it, only to gain it back again. I found myself cycling my weight gain and weight loss for six years as I went through four pregnancies. I used to be a slender 135 pounds, but found myself at 250 pounds, ugh! Not being able to ride bikes or go sledding with my children made me realize I had to change.

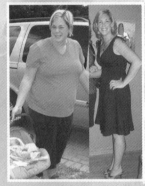

BEFORE   AFTER

I sat in my first Maximized Living Makeover with my eyes wide open. It was the most life-changing information I ever heard. I have radically transformed my diet, and I even manage to make it to the gym four to five days a week as well. The most important transformation was not just for me but my children. Having to raise four kids sometimes leaves them with the easiest meals. Hot dogs, Kraft dinners, and Eggo waffles were popular in my household. Making "adult" meals only meant leftovers that I would eventually pick away at. However, we made the transition and, slowly but surely, the kids got used to the green things adults call "cucumbers." The most important thing is that I am a role model for my children and thrive on watching them live a healthier lifestyle. Believe it or not, for all the skeptical mothers out there who dread the food fights they know they will have to endure with their own children during the changes that need to be made, they will come around a lot faster than you think!

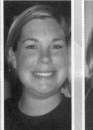 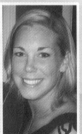

I have lost over one hundred pounds and plan on never going back. Thank you Maximized Living for helping us transform into a Maximized family.

BEFORE   AFTER

CHAPTER 3

Step One Toward the Cruise Ship
A Maximized Mind Is Your Secret Weapon

*"Men occasionally stumble over the truth,
but most of them pick themselves up and
hurry off as if nothing ever happened."[1]*

—*Sir Winston Churchill*

Special Note From Coauthor
By Dr. Charles Majors

ABOUT TWO MONTHS AGO, THERE was a woman in the front row of my Maximized Living Makeover who had a whole lot of beliefs that were holding her back. She was about 20 pounds overweight and believed there was no way she was going to be able to lose the weight. She was already on two medications and believed she was going to be on those medications for the rest of her life. She believed she didn't have enough time to work out. She believed there was no way she could afford to eat healthily. She believed her husband would never want to follow a new lifestyle.

Have you ever had some of those same beliefs? Do you believe some of those things right now? Fortunately, after hearing me talk, this woman was willing to challenge some of those beliefs and to begin following the protocols we teach. Within one month she lost 10 pounds, found the time to work out, and saw how easy it was to afford healthy food. She came off both of her medications, and best of all, her husband began seeing her changes. Now he believes and also started working out and following a Maximized Living lifestyle.

Do You Have Beliefs That Limit You?
Ask yourself:

- Have you ever started a diet on Monday and quit by Tuesday?

- Have you ever signed up for a gym membership, worked out for a few weeks, and then stopped?

- Have you ever bought a book, started reading it, and now you don't even know where that book is?

- Have you ever tried to lose weight and just quit because it wasn't happening fast enough?

- Do you believe that you are too old to lose weight?

- Do you believe that you will be on medications forever?

- Do you believe that because your mom is overweight that you will be too?

- Do you believe that you can't afford to eat well?

- Do you believe that your spouse will never change?

- Do you believe you can't change or overcome your circumstances?

If you said yes to any of these questions, then you have a limiting belief. A limiting belief is a belief you have formed in your mind that is stopping you from making progress.

You may be asking, "How do I know if I have any limiting beliefs?" The clue that you have a belief holding you back is the simple fact that you are not making any sustained progress in areas of your life that are important to you. It could be your weight, health, finances, relationships, work, and so on.

> If you change your beliefs, you change your behavior and it gets easy.

For example: Let's say you set a goal to lose 25 pounds, so you start eating better and exercising every day. In only a few weeks you step on the scale and you've lost five pounds, you look better in the mirror and everyone begins to notice your changes! Yet, soon you start skipping exercise, eating more desserts, and your new clothes stop fitting well. Rather than getting back to work, you ask yourself, "Why is this happening?" Or you say, "Here we go again."

You go on a diet and start losing weight, and the next thing you know you "fall off the wagon." But you didn't fall off of anything. You have a belief somewhere inside of you that says, "You'll never be skinny," "You're too lazy," or "You never stick to anything," and your subconscious mind says, "You're right!" Out come the Oreos, and you stay the same. You don't have an eating problem, exercise problem, or money problem. You have a belief problem, and that's what we are about to change. That is the secret weapon of all of our patients who have made such incredible lasting changes that were easy. If you change your beliefs, you change your behavior and it gets easy.

Testimonial — *Bryon Bella, 35 years old*

New Beliefs, New Habits

There are many things in life that rob us of our potential to be the complete person that we were created to be, and many of those things are addictions. Ever since I was eight years old, food has been my best friend, but it has robbed me of the person I was meant to be. I realize now that's no friend at all. Recently I took a long, hard look at that relationship and admitted to myself that it was not working out. I was addicted to food, and I could no longer enjoy life the way I used to. I'd tried to lose weight before, and when they say old habits die hard, they sure aren't kidding. I have probably lost and regained over 500 pounds throughout my entire lifetime.

Maximized Living has changed my entire life. I have lost over 90 pounds and the weight keeps coming off. Maximized Living has changed my belief system about who I really am, and helped me understand why I was eating in the first place. With a new level of thinking about myself came new action steps that carried me beyond the bad habits. If you don't change your belief system, you'll never change your habits!

Many of you are just like me, and we need to find the causes behind what drives us to turn to food. I had replaced people with food because it didn't judge me or disappoint me the way people did. I had used food to comfort me in pain and loneliness, as well as to celebrate every success. There was no

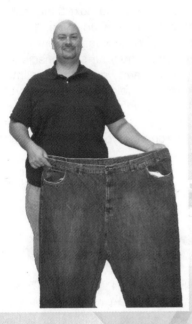

occasion unaccompanied by food. Now, however, I am recognizing these patterns and I am starting to talk myself into better decisions. I must reason with myself and ask people around me to show me when I am blind to my own poor choices. I can do all of these things with Maximized Living because it contains the elements to being a healthier person inside and out. Maximized Living has shown me that I have the help I need in seminars, my personal chiropractic appointments, and classes that encourage me to keep digging deeper and discover the healthy person inside of me. Now I'm using those tools every day and discovering health that has helped me live a more fulfilling life.

Testimonial – *Carol Kratz, 45 years old*

Yes I Can

I feel like I have been told, "You can't," my entire life. I have been over-weight ever since I was a child, and I feel like it had been just a way of life for me. I remember being teased when I was younger and how that has effected how I feel about my weight for years. My entire family, including my father, mother, and sister have struggled with our health and weight for many years. I remember my mother telling me that we had bad genes and that being "big-boned" was what our family was cursed with. I remember telling myself, "Well, I guess that's just the way it is."

It wasn't until Maximized Living that I changed my entire life. It taught me that I could change my life and gave me the inspiration to succeed and see me for who I really was—a person who was healthy, vibrant, and capable.

When I started getting help from Maximized Living, I noticed that I felt more energetic and wanted to move rather than lounge in front of the TV. I began to listen to my body more. It told me to make healthy choices, to choose carrots and celery over chips and cookies, and to drink water instead of soda or juice. I followed its advice, and I now completely follow all the Five Essentials of Maximized Living. As a result, I have lost over 100 pounds. I used to think I would be fat all my life, as if I had a genetic curse. Now I know I can control my own health. This program has drastically changed my life, and I am eternally grateful. With the support of the Maximized Living team, I know I can stay on this journey toward a healthier, more fulfilling life.

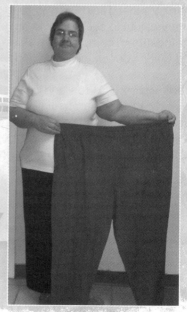

Your Big Why

If a person has a big enough Why, they can endure almost any how.
We want you to meet Team Hoyt, made up of father, Dick, and son, Rick. You may have seen them on TV. They have done over one thousand marathons and triathlons together. That's pretty impressive, but what is really impressive is the oxygen. Rick was diagnosed as a Spastic Quadriplegic with Cerebral Palsy from birth. At age nine, Ricky asked his dad if he would push him in his wheelchair in a five-mile run. Dick couldn't run up five steps without breathing hard, much less five miles. But because he loves his son, he decided to start jogging to start getting in shape. They completed the five miles and finished next to last. That night, Rick said, "Dad, when I'm running, it feels like I'm not handicapped." The rest is history.

When they do Ironman Triathlons, Dick now swims over two miles, pulling Ricky behind him in a boat. He then harnesses his son on a special bike and rides 100 miles in the blazing heat before pushing Ricky 26 miles. That's quite a change from someone who was overweight and couldn't go up the stairs without being out of breath.

If you ask why he performs a triathlon and does the work of two triathletes, he'll tell you it's because of the smile he sees on his son's face when they finish together. Dick's Why is strong enough that he will endure pain and suffering, just to see the smile on his son's face when they cross the finish line together. The bond they share goes way beyond words. It has been said that if your why is strong enough, you can bear almost any how.

Dick knew how to run and swim, he just never had a big enough why. You have the same potential inside of you as Team Hoyt; you just need a bigger why. It may be seeing your grandkids grow up, proving your doctor wrong, or any number of things, but it needs to be big enough so that you will do whatever it takes to make it happen.

"My Big Why"

Special Note from Coauthor Dr. Eric Shuemake

I've been someone who has struggled with eating right for most of my life. I was brought up on junk food. I had a steady diet of the three Ds – Dr. Pepper, Doritos, and do-nuts – for the first 20 years of my life. I was taught to eat these "comfort foods" when things got stressful. Once I started taking nutrition classes in college and learning how bad these things are for you, I still had problems staying away from them.

That all changed about ten years ago when I watched my grandmother die from the complications of diabetes. She died a miserable death because of the food choices she made. She was on dialysis three days a week for the last five years of her life. She was on so much medication that her liver started to shut down. She gained 50 pounds of water weight and became so swollen that you could hardly recognize her. By the time she died, she was on 25 drugs and they made her hallucinate so badly that she didn't recognize her own children and grandchildren next to her bed. The last few weeks of her life cost her almost half-a-million dollars in hospital bills. Because of the poor lifestyle choices she made, my grandmother was terrified and broke when she died.

My Why got really big, really fast, when I saw what it all did to my mom. The stress of taking care of my grand-mother almost killed my mom. One day I decided that I would never do that to my children. They would never have to take care of me while I wasted away and died. I would never spend the money that I was supposed to leave to them on being sick. Once that became my rea-son for eating well, things became easy. I no longer want-ed the three Ds. Now I have the best diet of just about anyone I know. The only thing that changed was my why!

Day 2 of the challenge will help you determine your BIG WHY.

Testimonial — *Bob Dillenger, 50 years old*

A Real Father Figure

T ime sure does fly. Before I knew it, I was turning fifty and had a grandson. I felt fine and didn't take any daily meds. Although I'd put on a little weight over the years, neither my wife nor I could lose it for long. I figured we all carry some extra padding at that age, so when my fifty-year physical came due, I wasn't worried.

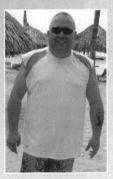

I walked in, and right away the nurse announced I'd be leaving with a prescription for high blood pressure. That was the first surprise. Next, the test for cholesterol came back high, and then my blood sugar turned up borderline. So from one day to the next, I had three chronic conditions, with three daily prescriptions they said I would have to take for the rest of my life. Suddenly, I really felt old. Fortunately, friends suggested that there was another way and invited my wife and me to a Maximized Living Seminar dinner. The presenter's advice about how to get healthy and get off my pills made sense to me. But more than that, he started me thinking about my goals in life.

First I realized that I hated the idea of being on medication. I had always been healthy until now. Was this inevitable? I decided I wanted to live as long as I could.

Second I really wanted to lose that extra weight. Not only did I want to be more attractive to my wife, but I also dreamed of retiring in good health, traveling, and enjoying time with her. I wondered if I would be able to do that.

Most importantly, I recognized that I wanted to be there for my grandson. I grew up without a father figure. When I watched others celebrating the men in their lives, I could only guess how it must have felt. I wanted to set an example as a good man for my grandson and son-in-law. For me that meant being healthy enough to take my grandson fishing and play outdoor games with him. I wanted to watch him grow with my encouragement and unconditional love.

I'm not complaining. I have received much more than I expected in life. To show my appreciation for what I have learned, I want to be a better man and a positive influence on my family, at work, in church, and with my friends. So I started to follow the Maximized Living plan of eating better and surge training.

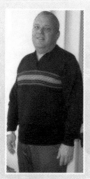

At first I didn't think I had the willpower to follow the Advanced Eating Plan. How could I give up sugar and bread, two things I loved to eat? But I saw my friend do it, and I decided to try. I started at 225 pounds with a 40 inch waist. For three months I stayed on the diet, intending to lose 30 pounds before my wife and I went on vacation. On the Sunday before we left, the scale read 190. I haven't made other goals yet, but I mean to make these changes permanent. So far, it's been a lot easier than I thought.

CHAPTER 4

Why You Can't Lose Weight
*What You Don't Know Will Hurt You,
or at Least Keep You Fat*

---

*"Education is learning what you didn't
even know you didn't know."[1]*

—*Daniel J. Boorstin*
(American social historian and educator, 1914)

THERE ARE DOZENS OF POPULAR nutrition and weight-loss programs that rely on their own brand of snack bars, meal replacement shakes, and supplements. If you read the label on most of those products, you'll find that they contain damaged fats, neurotoxic artificial sweeteners like Sucralose and Aspartame, and other ingredients that make you sick. They may help you lose weight, but you will only die lighter and make carrying your coffin easier on your pallbearers. It won't delay the funeral at all!

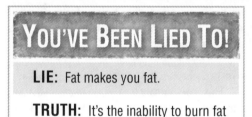

YOU'VE BEEN LIED TO!

LIE: Fat makes you fat.

TRUTH: It's the inability to burn fat that makes you fat.

The fat-free era was arguably the worst era in the history of nutrition. While bad fats should be avoided, good fats are critical to health, leanness, and well-being. You need fats for brain function, cell structure and function, and your glands need fat for balanced hormone production. Fats also supply insulation and protection for your organs, help store and transport fat-soluble vitamins (A, D, E, and K), assist in mineral absorption, reduce hunger signals, and slow food absorption, which will allow for better blood sugar control, glandular activity, and weight loss. As far as making you fat, fats are actually needed to mobilize and burn fat. So really, no "good" fat makes you fat!

Understanding Weight-Loss Resistance

Can you relate to this? You go to the gym and sweat on the stair stepper for an hour several days a week and don't seem to be looking a whole lot leaner or thinner. Or you go out to lunch with your co-workers and eat a "smart lunch" while they all eat hamburgers. Meanwhile, they look great (don't you hate those people!) and your lettuce seems to be going right to your stomach and thighs.

You try to watch your diet, buy diet books and exercise equipment, and try all kinds of programs, but you still can't lose any real weight or get your body firm in the right places. If that's you or a version of you, we have good news. You don't have to struggle anymore. We know your problem. You are weight-loss resistant (WLR). One of the key problems causing WLR is a hormone called Leptin. Your brain is no longer hearing it, and we've helped thousands of people overcome this. Look at what happens when you get this important hormone under control.

Tuning Out Leptin

One key reason that so many people (and probably you) are weight-loss resistant is an imbalance in a hormone called Leptin. Leptin was discovered recently and is the hormone that tells your brain to burn fat. If you have normal levels of Leptin, your brain gets the signal, you burn fat, and have no problem keeping your ideal weight. When weight-loss resistance happens, you have too much Leptin in your body.

Think of Leptin as your mother-in-law. Now, if she is constantly yelling at you, what are you going to do? Put your fingers in your ears and tune her out. The same thing happens when your Leptin is constantly in the system. It's screaming, "Burn fat! Burn fat! Burn fat!" to your brain all day long and eventually your brain just tunes it out. The "burn fat" signal is no longer heard.

Your past habits have caused you to hit a wall, and your current habits are ineffective because of your hormones.

The answer isn't more Leptin. The body is producing it. The brain just isn't listening, so the Leptin stops working. In fact, the result of this is that you actually end up with a whole lot of Leptin in your system, but the body is now desensitized to it and it no longer works to burn fat. This is exactly what you are dealing with now. Because of past habits that allowed for too much fat in the system, you went to the Leptin well too often. Now, no matter how many calories you count or how much you exercise, you will not burn fat. Your past habits have caused you to hit a wall, and your current habits are ineffective because of your hormones.

To fix your hormone problem, you have to address your ineffective, elevated Leptin levels.

Two Key Lifestyle Factors to Address to Improve This Hormone Problem

One of the main factors to improving the hormone function in your body is to stop eating too many grains and sugars (this is 90 percent of Americans). This gives you problems with two hormones—Insulin and Leptin. With too many grains and sugars, the hormone insulin stops working and so you keep storing sugar as fat. Too much fat and you get the ineffective, elevated Leptin issue. This goes on until the whole fat-burning process stops working!

The second factor is lowering cellular toxicity (which we will discuss later in the book in step four). Because of issues related to hormones, many people have become the opposite of what they want to be – a fat-building, muscle-burning machine. In step two, "Lose Ten Pounds Fast," the goal is to begin turning you back into what you were supposed to be – a fat-burning, muscle-building machine.

Soon, you'll become more like one of those people you hate, who tend to stay lean and thin, versus someone who tends to stay the opposite. In fact, becoming a fat burner will not just make you look better and weigh less, but it will also radically alter your life and future. As a matter of fact, Ron Rosedale, MD, nutrition and metabolic expert and author of The Rosedale Diet, says: "Health and life span is determined by the propor-tion of fat versus sugar people burn throughout their lifetime. The more fat you burn as fuel, the healthier you will be. The more sugar you burn as fuel, the more disease-ridden you will be and the shorter your life will likely be."[2]

If you are reading this, chances are that you are a sugar burner and we are going to change that. The "Lose Ten Pounds Fast" plan also gets to the heart of 99 percent of chronic disease in this country: inflammation. That brings us to one more lie you need to destroy before you start losing ten pounds.

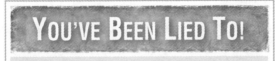

YOU'VE BEEN LIED TO!

LIE: Cholesterol causes heart disease.

TRUTH: Inflammation causes heart disease.

Testimonial – *James Shelley, 38 years old, and family*

Cruise Ship, Here I Come

I never knew that my weight problem was actually a hormone problem! I had tried everything and was never able to lose any weight until I found out how to get my Leptin levels under control. Before starting the program, I suffered from daily fatigue, soreness, and sleep apnea. I was tired all the time, so I never felt like exercising. As a result, my weight was steadily

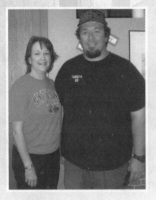

increasing. Being sick and overweight was costing me a lot of joy in my life. My job was harder, and I hated watching my health go downhill.

Under the Maximized Living program, I got spinal adjustments, detoxification, and I followed the Lose Ten Pounds Fast eating plan. I also began surge training. I lost more than ten pounds though. I lost 40 pounds in two months! With the great recipes, it was a breeze. This is the first time I've ever been able to keep weight off because my Leptin imbalance is fixed. By continuing my surge training just twelve minutes a week, it's been almost effortless to keep it off.

I realized my neck was in terrible shape when I learned about the Arc of Life and how much it controls organ function and health. Now I know that being adjusted will be a part of the rest of my life. Each treatment feels as if it turns the lights on in the areas of my body that have degenerated. I had surgery a few years ago, and they botched the epidural, leaving me with numbness and burning in my legs when I was on my feet. Since I started getting the power turned on, that is gone! I never thought that it would go away, and it feels great to know that I can heal. I lay hardwood floors for a living, and the other guys are having a hard time keeping up with me now.

I love how I feel, but Maximized Living has been a huge blessing for my family too. My wife lived for a long time with depression, seasonal allergies, and neck and back pain. She had tried drugs and other chiropractors without success. On the Advanced Eating Plan, she lost 12 pounds quickly. She sleeps much better now and has enough energy to keep up with our kids!

Our sons are also benefiting from adjustments and a better diet. The older one is doing well in school without his ADD medicine, and our youngest is able to control his behavior better and is no longer wetting the bed at night.

I have more energy than I've had in years, and I know that I will be regenerating instead of degenerating for the rest of my life. You will find me on that cruise ship!

The idea that fat in our diet is the reason for our current epidemic of heart disease came about when it was observed that the plaques in the arteries of heart attack patients contained fat and cholesterol. The Framingham Study, which began in 1948 and continued for many years, was designed to prove "the lipid hypothesis."[3] The lipid hypothesis is the theory that there is a direct relationship between your chance of having a heart attack, and the amount of saturated fat (animal fat) and cholesterol in your diet.

The Framingham Study followed 5,000 people and checked on them every five years. People who consumed large amounts of animal fat and cholesterol were compared with those who consumed very little. After years of study, Dr. William Castelli finally admitted, "In Framingham, Massachusetts the more saturated fat one ate, the more cholesterol one ate, the more calories one ate, the lower the person's serum cholesterol. We found that the people who ate the most cholesterol, ate the most saturated fat, and ate the most calories, weighed the least and were the most active."[4]

The years of study found that cholesterol was not predictive of heart attack at all after the age of forty-seven. In other words, once a man reaches the age of 48, there is no relationship between high levels of cholesterol and dying of heart attack.

If that's not clear enough, check out this quote from another researcher in the study, Dr. George V. Mann: "The diet-heart hypothesis has been repeatedly shown to be wrong, and yet, for complicated reasons of pride, profit, and prejudice, the hypothesis continues to be exploited by scientists, fund-raising enterprises, food companies, and even governmental agencies. The public is being deceived by the greatest health scam of the century."[5]

Again, you are being lied to! Look at the TV. The commercials say that these drugs lower your risk of a heart attack, right? Well, on the Crestor commercial, at the bottom of the screen, it tells you that Crestor hasn't been determined to lower your risk of heart attack. Here it is from their Web site: "Crestor has not been approved to prevent heart disease, heart attack, or stroke."[6] Look it up.

Lying with Statistics

British Prime Minister, Benjamin Disraeli once said, "There are three kinds of lies: lies, damned lies, and statistics." [7] Television ads for Lipitor featuring artificial heart inventor Dr. Robert Jarvik, (who never practiced medicine), claims that Lipitor will lower heart attack risk by 36 percent.[8]

Sounds great, right? Let's look at the fine print. Where do they get those numbers? "In a large clinical study, three percent of people taking a placebo had a heart attack and two percent of those taking Lipitor had a heart attack."[9]

Let's do the math.

For every 100 people in the trial that lasted three-and-a-half years, three people on the placebo and two people on Lipitor had heart attacks. That is one less heart attack for every one hundred people. In other words, 100 people had to take Lipitor for three-and-a-half years to prevent one heart attack. What this really means is that 99 out of one hundred people taking Lipitor received no benefit.

Dr. Jerome R. Hoffman, Professor of Clinical Medicine at UCLA, put it this way: "What if you put 250 people in a room and told them they would have to pay over $1,000 per year for a medicine they must take every day that might give them diarrhea and muscle pain, and that 249 of those people would get no benefit? How many would take that?"[10]

So what is the true cause of heart disease?

Inflammation of your arteries. It does matter what you eat, but that is not what you've been taught. The key is reducing inflammation in your arteries. We will show you how to do that by changing the fats you eat, not reducing them. Many of you will need to add anti-inflammatory fats to your diet, and that is good news because the fats we will tell you to eat taste really good. Eating a low-fat melba toast and celery diet just doesn't work. Since the low-fat craze began, heart disease has skyrocketed in this country, and it's time to stop it in its tracks from destroying your future and your family.

CHAPTER 5

Step Two Toward the Cruise Ship
Lose Twenty Pounds Fast

"Everyone has inside himself a piece of good news!
The good news is that you really don't know how great
you can be, how much you can love, what you can
accomplish, and what your potential is!"[1]

— Anne Frank

REMEMBER, IT'S NOT WHERE YOU stand right now that matters; it's where you're going. You have more potential in you than you will ever know. Many of you have bought into the myth that you can't lose weight and keep it off, or that it has to be hard. You probably believe that because you've experienced a lot of losses in the weight-loss battle and not a lot of wins. Step two, "Lose Twenty Pounds Fast," is designed to get you a win. In this step we will tell you what to eat, how to make it, and how to exercise so that you lose at least ten pounds quickly. In our offices, this process takes anywhere from a week to a month.

Your Secret Weight-Loss Weapon
By Dr. Ben Lerner

Thinking Your Way Into a Better Future

I have three children—one teenager and two under the age of ten. When my son hit his teenage years, I discovered a major limiting belief. I was of the mind that the teenage years were seven years of bad luck and that I was just someone who couldn't communicate well or have a good time with teenagers. I believed we didn't have that much in common and that I just didn't understand them.

Thankfully, it occurred to me—what kind of strategy is that? With one teenager and two on the way, I'd doomed myself to a bad relationship with all of my children. No wonder some people keep having babies; they're cute when they're puppies.

You literally think your way into your future. If I decided to have trouble with teenagers, then I was creating a troubled future. With that in mind, I changed my limiting belief of "I don't get along with teenagers" to "Right now, I look, feel, and act like a teenager and can have fun and talk for hours with my son and his friends."

That's a much more intelligent mind-set and a far better strategy for thinking my way into a peaceful, successful future.

> You literally think your way into your future

If you change from "I don't like exercise," "I love bread," "I'm a sugar-aholic," "I can't," or "I always quit these things," to "I love the feeling of satisfaction after I exercise," "I love the fact that I can add all of these great fats for good taste and get fuller easier," "I won't miss the sugar," and "I love doing everything I can to live longer, have energy, and be alive and a role model for my family," then you're adopting a way better strategy for the future!

We know you've tried diet and exercise plans before, but what happened? You didn't stick to the plan. You are fixing that with your new secret weapon! Refer to the Maximized Mind Exercises every day for 30 days to reprogram your limiting beliefs into empowering beliefs. Until you transform your beliefs about you, your ability, your opportunity to transform, and how easy it will be to continue this for the rest of your life, you won't change. Through a Maximized Mind, you're going to quickly abandon your limiting beliefs for abundant, empowering ones.

Testimonial – *Vivian Shuemake, 57 years old*

Making It Work

My mother had diabetes by the time she was 35, so when I reached 50 and didn't have it, I thought I'd dodged the bullet. A year later, I was diagnosed with it as well. I was just learning about the Maximized Living principles, so I decided to put them to the test. One month after starting the eating plan, my blood sugar was normal. I've struggled with my weight for about 25 years, so I was delighted

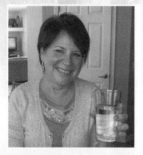

when the pounds started to go. I've lost 35 pounds since then. I wish I'd measured the inches, but I've gone from an extra large to a medium and it feels wonderful!

I ate the recipes that you'll find in this book. The eating plan guide is great for those of you who want it all spelled out, but I like a little less structure. If you're like me, you won't drink a smoothie if you want eggs and that's OK. Change it around to suit you, and you'll be just fine. I love leftovers and used those often in place of a new meal. The secret to success is planning, shopping, and cooking. Always have at least one of these recipes ready to go so you won't reach for a frozen pizza or stop at a fast food restaurant when your schedule gets thrown off. If you have the proper food in the house, preferably cooked and in the fridge, you won't eat the bad stuff. If you stay on it faithfully with no cheating, the cravings will be gone in about seven to ten days. I didn't believe that I would ever not want sugar, potatoes, or pasta, but I don't! I can walk around plates of donuts and brownies all day and not eat one. You're going to feel so much better that you won't want to go back to bad eating habits.

I'm 57 and feel better than I have in 20 years. I want to dance at my grand-children's weddings, go to my son's silver wedding anniversary party, and go somewhere wonderful with my daughter and her husband for her 60th birthday. I have no doubt I'll achieve these goals by staying on the principles. If I can do it, anyone can!

Secret To Losing Twenty Pounds Fast:
The Advanced Eating Plan

Eating this way rapidly attacks issues with your hormones, like Insulin and Leptin, to help you overcome weight-loss resistance and cause you to become a fat-burning machine. Improving hormones and eating the foods on this plan also goes after inflammation like a heat-seeking missile. Because of this, many people see their blood pressure go down, triglycerides decrease, and arthritis pain go down. Decreasing inflammation slows down the aging process. We hear people say that they sleep better, have more energy, and feel younger just by starting the eating plan.

We are going to attack those hormone issues starting right now. Here are the guidelines for the next seven to thirty days, depending on how long it takes you to lose ten pounds. You don't have to remember everything, just follow the eating plan included in this chapter and the recipes in the 28 day challenge.

Here are five eating guidelines for losing twenty pounds fast:
1. Eliminate sugars.
2. Cut out grains.
3. Remove bad fats and add good fats.
4. Consume very little fruit.
5. Avoid toxins.

Guideline 1: Eliminate Sugars

Eliminate all sugars and everything that turns to sugar. This is the key to the Lose Twenty Pounds Fast Plan. We would like to stress that this is not a high-protein or low-carb diet. You are loading up on quality proteins, good fats, and vegetables, not just eating whatever you want as long as it's not a carb. The type of eating you're going to do here is necessary to heal your Insulin and Leptin issues.

Remember, the Insulin and Leptin receptors are fried from all the sugar and fat in your system. The goal is to metabolically shift your body from burning sugar to burning fat. Being a sugar burner is why you get cravings for sweets or bread products. Your brain is telling you to eat sugar so that it has something to burn. The only way to get your body to switch into fat-burning mode is to get off the sugar so that you repair the Insulin and Leptin receptors. And the only way to do that is by eliminating sugar until the receptors are healed.

When your receptors are healed, your body will start to "hear" the signals again so you can stop producing so much fat and start burning the fat you have. At this point, you will even burn fat in your sleep, the way you were designed. Plus, the sugar cravings and your addiction to carbohydrates go away.

NOTE: Since your body is only burning sugar right now, how do you think you may feel the first day or so that you eliminate sugar? Tired, cranky, and sluggish? Yes, and that is a sign that you are healing and switching into fat-burning mode. After that, it's easy and you have more energy than you've ever had. When your body goes into fat-burning mode, it literally uses your unwanted fat to fuel your furnace. It's a vicious circle finally working in your favor. Ultimately, you'll burn more fat, preserve muscle, and you'll have more energy to do the things you haven't been able to do. Soon, you won't really want the sugar anymore (or at least the sugar monster will roar softer). That's the magic!

How to Remove All Sugars and Everything That Turns to Sugar from Your Diet

Sugar is an "antinutrient." It offers no significant amounts of vitamins and minerals and, in fact, actually robs your body of precious nutrient stores. This inevitably can only fast track you down the road of popular new millennium diseases such as chronic fatigue, ADD, ADHD, heart disease, diabetes, and cancers and make you susceptible to infections like colds and flus.

Americans consume an average of 120 pounds of sugar per year, per person. Compare this to only five pounds per year, per family in the early 1900s. These sugars are hidden in virtually every boxed food, cereal, and cracker. Even some fruit juices labeled "100 percent juice" typically contain more sugar than a can of soda.

> Some fruit juices labeled "100 percent juice" typically contain more sugar than a can of soda.

High glycemic foods, particularly refined sugars, unnaturally and aggressively elevate Insulin and Leptin. Prolonged spiking and elevation of Insulin and Leptin lead to Insulin and Leptin resistance and, as we've mentioned, ultimately causes weight-loss resistance. This also leads to premature aging, emotional disturbances that can lead to depression, type 2 diabetes, and inflammation that leads to conditions like heart disease (inflammation of the arteries) and cancer.

Removing processed grains and refined sugars seems tough because they are everywhere. Yes, this includes white rice, white pasta, and white bread. These are processed grains that turn into "sugar" and raise Glucose and Insulin the same as sucrose, fructose, or any other "-ose."

One-third of sugar consumption comes from soft drinks, while two-thirds of our sugar intake comes from hidden sources, including lunch meats, pizza, sauces, breads, soups, crackers, fruit drinks, canned foods, yogurt, ketchup, and mayonnaise.

The following are sweeteners you need to avoid like the plague. They are present in many packaged foods:
- Sugar
- Aspartame (Nutrasweet)
- Sucralose (Splenda)
- Corn syrup
- High fructose corn syrup

Removing all refined sugar is probably the hardest of the changes because most Americans are addicted to sugary foods. To our bodies, sugar is an addictive drug like cocaine. If there is any lingering doubt of this fact, just talk to someone who gave up sugar and experienced classic detox symptoms like headaches, shakes, gastrointestinal trouble, fatigue, and mood swings. These symptoms alone should serve as a warning about how dangerous sugar is to the body.

Experience has shown that it takes about one week for cravings for sugar and breads to cease. Any indulgence in sugar during this time, no matter how small, will trigger cravings. Therefore, we recommend an "all-or-nothing" approach to sugar.

Testimonial – *Judy Stephens, 69 years old*
What Sugar Cravings?

Before I found Maximized Living, I took at least 13 pills every single day for my high blood pressure, acid reflux, allergies, osteoporosis, high cholesterol, low blood calcium, and thyroid cancer. I had drugs to cover up the side effects of the other drugs! I was the sort of person that made drug companies rich. My brain felt so foggy that I struggled to stay awake when I was driving. I was hurting so much in my joints that I couldn't run my business. I was overweight and had tried everything—diet books, exercise programs, you name it. After working out for two years with my husband, I actually gained weight! Nothing was working until I found Maximized Living.

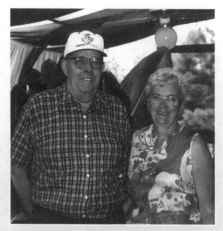

I decided to start the Maximized Living program and I'm glad I did. Right away after receiving my first adjustment, I slept a lot better. My husband and I began the Advanced Eating Plan and took up surge training, riding a recumbent bike at home three days a week. I then got rid of all the toxins that were making us sick. My biggest source of toxins was the pills I'd taken for so long.

The results have been amazing. I lost 30 pounds in three months, something I was never able to do in three years before! Jim lost 40 pounds in the same three months. He had been diagnosed with COPD and was on multiple medications, which he no longer has to take. At first it was hard to eliminate sugar and all the foods that turn to sugar, which I craved. But I learned how to overcome the cravings by just giving my body what it needs and not through sheer will power. The cravings went away, and we don't look or feel like the same people!

Now that I am eating and living well, I have found that I actually don't need all those pills I was taking. My blood pressure is normal, my acid reflux is gone, my cholesterol is normal, and my allergies have cleared up. I'm no longer a slave to my drugs! I have gotten off of every one, except for thyroid medications that I take two times a week instead of every day.

We were able to quit the gym because we do surge training at home, saving us money and giving us more time to do the things we love. I have more energy than I've had in years, so I'm able to enjoy my hobby of gardening a lot more. Best of all, I know I will live longer and better as long as I keep on maximizing my health.

Guideline 2: Cut Out the Grains

No grains, not even whole grains, are allowed because they turn to sugar. During the Lose Twenty Pounds Fast phase, this is extremely important. Just follow the food guide and recipes we've given you, and your body will do the rest. Once weight loss is no longer an issue, you can start to add some healthy, whole grains back in to your diet, such as:

- Barley
- Buckwheat
- Millet
- Semolina
- Tapioca
- Cereals
- Wheat crackers
- Whole-grain tortillas

- Brown rice
- Bulgar (tabouli)
- Rye
- Steel cut oats
- Whole-grain breads
- Whole grains
- Ezekiel bread
- Spelt

Guideline 3: Remove Bad Fats and Add Good Fats

Remove bad fats such as hydrogenated and partially hydrogenated oils, trans fats, and rancid vegetable oils. These are linked to cellular congestion leading to cancer, chronic fatigue, and neurotoxic syndrome. Bad fats are also linked to chronic inflammation, which is the key to twenty-first-century medicine. Heart disease, stroke, cancer, diabetes, and other diseases are the leading causes of death in the United States, and inflammation is at the root.

Add good fats from Olive Oil, Coconut Oil, flax, avocado, fish, or healthy meats. Good fats are the most lacking nutrient in the Standard American Diet (SAD), not vitamins and minerals. Remember, you actually need good fats to burn fat.

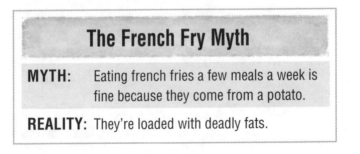

The French Fry Myth

MYTH: Eating french fries a few meals a week is fine because they come from a potato.

REALITY: They're loaded with deadly fats.

The half-life of trans fats or hydrogenated fats is fifty-one days. This means that after fifty-one days, only half of the negative effects of this man-made fat have been processed. The body needs fifty-one additional days, or a total of 102 days, to remove the majority of the trans fats and their negative effects, such as decreased nerve transmission, decreased focus, and an increase in hyperactivity. Other negative effects include decreased immunity and an increased risk of cancer, diabetes, and heart disease.

As you can see, not all fats are automatically bad for you. In fact, your body needs fats, but it needs the right ones.

Probably the biggest question we get about fats is "does it matter what kind of fish oil or omega oils I take?" Our answer is a resounding yes. Essential fatty acid supplements like fish oil are an incredible way to decrease inflammation, boost your immune system and improve your moods, but only if your body can use them. Research shows that your body works best when the essential fatty acids are in a certain ratio. That's why many people consume fish oil supplements, but don't see the benefits. For that reason, we recommend **Perfect Ratio Omega®** and 2 mg of the powerful Astaxanthin. A series of fatty acids are included in this supplement, derived from sources like Flaxseed Oil and fish oil. The latter has been shown to support healthy heart, brain, immune and joint function. Countries with the highest fish consumption also have the lowest rates of depression. There is evidence that it may reduce the risk of dementia and reduce the cognitive impairments associated with Alzheimer's disease. According to a UCLA study, Omega-3 supplements in fish oil can help the brain produce plaque fighting proteins used in preventing Alzheimer's.

Omega-3's are some of the good fats that are part of a healthy diet, but they are not produced by your body. Thus, you must consume them from external sources. The same is true of Omega-6 fatty acids found in Perfect Ratio omega. The combination of Omega-3 and Omega-6 fats produces the optimal ratio that your body needs. Plus, there are 2 mg of the powerful Carotenoid Antioxidant, Astaxanthin.

Immune function is improved by the antioxidant properties of Astaxanthan, which protect your body from free radical damage. A study in the February 2004 issue of Journal of Pharmacological studies discussed the effects of Astaxanthan with Ginko Biloba to treat asthma. Results showed that the therapy reduced T cell activation similar to two popular antihistamine drugs- Zyrtec and Astalin.

Last but not least, **Perfect Ratio Omega**® contains 125% of the RDA of Vitamin D you need and 2mg of the powerful Astaxanthin. This ensures that your bones stay strong while your joints heal. The science behind this product is second to none when it comes to essential fatty acid supplements. This is one that should be in almost everyone's daily routine.

Slam-Dunk Time

If you see those bad fats, then run far, far away because that stuff will literally kill you. Go get a trash can and walk to your pantry. Pull out any package of cookies, chips, or anything else in a box and look for those bad fat words. If you see them, slam-dunk them in the trash can. Don't donate them to someone or use them up because you spent "good money on them." Would you donate a bottle of Arsenic to someone or use it up because you spent money on it? I don't think so. Slam-dunk them now!

There, wasn't that fun? By slam-dunking the trash where it belongs, you have taken a huge step toward the front of the cruise ship line. You've eliminated the fats that cause inflammation and almost every disease known to man. Now, we need to add the right fats that reduce inflammation and heal your body.

Stock your kitchen with these healthy fats. Many grocery stores are starting to carry the fats listed in the table on the next page, but not all. Plan a monthly trip to a health food store or a natural grocer to stock up on what you need.

Cooking with Fats and Oils without Turning Good Fats into Bad Fats

For high heat: Use only Coconut Oil or Grapeseed Oil for frying. The best choice is Coconut Oil because of its superior flavor when frying food such as chicken. Olive Oil will turn rancid when heated above 120 degrees. If it smokes, it has already turned rancid.

For medium heat: To sauté foods, use Extra Virgin Olive Oil, Sesame Oil, Grapeseed Oil, Coconut Oil, or butter.

For baking: Butter, Coconut Oil, Sunflower, Safflower, or Olive Oil can be used in temperatures less than 325 degrees. In a hotter oven, only use butter or Coconut Oil. If coating a pan or cookie sheet, use only Coconut Oil or Grapeseed Oil.

Core Good Fats to Stock in Your Kitchen

- Grass-fed meat
- Avocado
- Coconut or coconut flakes
- Organic butter
- Cod Liver Oil
- Grapeseed Oil Vegenaise® (a mayonnaise replacement)
- Raw cheeses
- Extra Virgin Olive Oil, olives
- Full-fat Coconut Milk and oil
- Flaxseed Oil
- Full-fat raw milk
- Grapeseed Oil
- Full-fat plain yogurt
- Almond butter
- Eggs
- Canned sardines in oil or water
- Raw nuts and seeds: almonds, cashews, flax, hemp, pecans, pine nuts, macadamia, sesame, sunflower, walnuts, and the like

Guideline 4: Consume Very Little Fruit

Eat very little fruit. Only one cup of berries, a small Granny Smith apple, or half a grapefruit per day is permitted. The 20 in 30 eating plan in the challenge at the back of the book takes this rule into consideration.

Guideline 5: Avoid Toxins

Toxins not only can make you fat, but they also can keep you that way. Toxins bind to fat and make these fats difficult to lose. Avoid man-made foods, additives, preservatives, colorings, artificial sweeteners (aspartame, Splenda, saccharine), sodas, and fried foods. Going natural will have an immediate weight loss effect as you're putting in nutrients your body was designed to use.

It will take several days to lower insulin levels. In the meantime, high insulin levels can cause headaches and general blah feelings. Hang in there—it will go away and be replaced with more energy than you ever thought possible! Most people have no symptoms at all. If you are diabetic and on medication, monitor your glucose levels carefully. They will go down quickly and you may have to adjust your meds with your doctor's supervision.

Testimonial – *Arthur L. Durand, 75 years old*

I Reversed My Diabetes in Two Weeks!

Before I found Maximized Living, I had been diabetic for ten years. I weighed 260 pounds, and sleep apnea made me miserable. Due to my size 48 waist, I needed clothes so large I felt like I was wearing a tent. I was hooked up to a C-PAP machine to sleep, and my feet hurt so much from the diabetes that I had to wear special shoes for neuropathy (nerve pain). I tried special diets to control my diabetes but nothing ever worked. I was uncomfortable and discouraged.

The Maximized Living program began to change all of that. I got spinal adjustments, followed the Advanced Eating Plan and exercised by doing surge training. Right away I began losing a pound every three days and had lost over 20 pounds in two months. In seven months, I had taken off 60 pounds. I am still losing weight, and I have dropped to a size 40. I can wear normal clothes now!

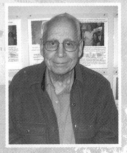

Even better, I am no longer diabetic! After only two weeks of starting the program, my morning (fasting) glucose level went from 229 (diabetic) to around 90-110 (normal). With few exceptions, it has stayed there for the last ten months.

Advanced Eating Plan Tips

1. Removing all grains and sugars is easiest when done cold turkey. In two to five days the cravings will be gone.

2. Eating more frequent meals will minimize symptoms related to glucose and insulin adjustments you may experience when removing grains and sugars. This also means no corn, which is a grain, and no potatoes of any kind, which are tubers, not vegetables.

3. Drink a lot of water—at least ten 8-ounce glasses a day.

4. Eat more vegetables! The ones that grow above ground. There's no limit to these.

5. Eliminate sugar, including corn syrup, fructose, honey, maltodextrin, dextrose, molasses, rice milk, fruit juices, maple syrup, dates, sugar cane, beet sugar, and lactose.

6. Sweeten with the herb Stevia, or use Xylitol.

7. The plate now has vegetables, fats, and proteins on it and not spaghetti, rice, cereal, or bread.

8. Stay full. Always keep something handy that is good for you to eat or make one of the smoothies, but don't get hungry. You must plan and prepare! Don't get caught at work or on the road without having brought plenty of the good things to eat!

IMPORTANT:

No matter how much of the good foods you're eating, you will most likely be Vitamin D deficient like 3 out of 4 Americans. The natural way humans get this vital nutrient occurs in the form of Vitamin D3 from the sun, but modern life and sun-related dangers don't allow us to get enough. It is generally recommended to start supplementing your diet with 5,000 IU a day. Taking **Vitamin D3 Complex**® supplement each day is equivalent to drinking 20 glasses of milk or eating 16 servings of fish! This supplement is also cultivated with antioxidants and nutrient-dense raw fruits and vegetables, and provides a very generous amount of probiotics.

Meal Times and Menus

Make a menu for each week. Sundays are the best time for many people. If you work, make meals ahead of time. Make enough for leftovers. Wash and bag veggies on Sunday for one week. They will stay fresh if you use vacuum bags with zip locks.

To add variety to your diet, find ten recipes that you like. If you rotate between only two or three meals, boredom will threaten your success. In the 28 day challenge in the back of the book, you will find more tips on meal planning, preparation and dining out.

For over one hundred great recipes, more great nutritional information, more meal plans, and more tips on how to follow the plans, you can buy the **Maximized Living Nutrition Plans**® book at a Maximized Living doctor's office or at **www.maximizedliving.com**.

YOU'VE BEEN LIED TO!

LIE: The wellness industry has been helping us get healthier and in better shape.

TRUTH: Most of today's nutrition guidance has been diluted down to the term "diet." This is due largely to the fact that people have gotten so large. With obesity on the increase, it's no wonder that when you talk about healthy eating, people think of the latest fad diet. The catch-22 is the health and diet industry is, in part, responsible for the current outrageous level of obesity!

CHAPTER 6

Step Three towards the cruise ship:
Become a fat burning machine!

Just look at what has happed since the "wellness" industry has taken off. It doesn't look like the "wellness" industry books have made us well, does it?

- Of all American adults, 61 percent are overweight.[2]

- One billion people worldwide are overweight, which Congress called "as serious a threat as global warming."[3]

- In the past 20 years, the number of overweight children ages six to eleven have doubled—tripled for adolescents.[4]

- The U.S. will have three new generations of degenerative illness in the near future.[5]

- A 22 pound weight gain (the average middle-age weight gain) increases heart attack risk by 75 percent. A 15 pound weight gain doubles your risk of developing type 2 diabetes.[6]

Testimonial – *Shelly Bracken, 35 years old*
Wisdom Is Better Than Gold

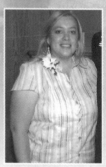

When I was at my heaviest weight (247 pounds), I would often wonder what I could possibly achieve or give back to others. I doubted that I had a real purpose or that I could leave a positive impact on this earth. With the physical and emotional struggles of obesity, I was trapped.

How can you feel positive about the future when you struggle to climb stairs or walk? I had no motivation, and I let my fears and insecurities hide behind my weight for years. I knew that I wanted to live the best life I could, but if you don't have your health, how can you do that?

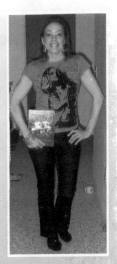

All the "low-fat" diet gimmicks always failed me and left me feeling like a failure. I would think, "If only I could start those pills...," "When I can buy that powder...," "When I start that new shake everyone's trying...," or "If I can just save up for those new products out now, then I can lose the weight." I was looking for the "gold," thinking that was the cure. It sometimes worked temporarily, but the gold would always run out, leaving me chasing more.

Discovering the Maximized Living Seminar finally gave me the wisdom to change my life. I lost the weight for good and watched my body heal as I removed the interferences to proper function.

Now I've lost over 90 pounds, and I'm staying at 130 pounds. If someone told me two-and-a-half years ago that this would be my life now, I would never have believed them. What is the secret?

Wisdom is better than gold. Take the time to learn the truth, and it will stay with you forever. You will never have to chase the gold again; you will never be duped, tricked, or seduced by it. This is my life now. No commercials or advertisements can pull me back. Nothing on TV or what others say can jeopardize my health. I am living my life the maximized way!

EXCUSE: "I don't have the time to exercise."

EXCUSE KILLER: The most effective exercise takes as little as 12 minutes per week!

You know, the craziest thing about time is that it seems to be lost. We just can't seem to find where time went. With the invention of more time- and labor-saving devices such as instant coffee, pay at the pump, ATMs, fast lanes both on the freeway and at the supermarket, and so on, you would think Americans would have too much time on our hands. On the contrary, we can't seem to find where time has gone.

How many of you really enjoy getting up before dawn and spending 45 minutes on the treadmill? Be honest! More than likely, you spend every single second on the treadmill wishing that the torture would be over! While 95 percent of the fitness gurus will have you believe that the effects of low-intensity classic aerobic exercise is the best way to burn body fat, the fact is that all that extra time on the stair-climber, stationary bike, rower, or treadmill may ultimately do more harm than good.

Research has now revealed that it's not simply what happens to you during the workout that matters; it's what happens afterward that ultimately makes the difference. While 30 to 40 minutes of jogging does improve cardiovascular function and burns a little fat during the session, research shows that after long, slow workouts Cortisol is increased. Cortisol is a hormone produced by stress on your system. This stress hormone actually increases fat storing and breaks down muscle. The exact opposite of what you want! If you go to the gym, you may have noticed that many of the regulars on the cardio equipment or in the classes have the exact same body type year after year. There is a reason for that and you're going to learn how to avoid it.

> All the extra time on the stair-climber, stationary bike, rower, or treadmill may ultimately do more harm than good.

You can regulate Cortisol and support your Glucose levels with **Max Fit®**, a fitness formula that will help you lose weight, build muscle, improve endurance, and increase energy while simultaneously helping to calm you. This supplement contains extracts of the herb Ashwaganda and decaffeinated green coffee bean as well as Carnitine and Creatine. Ask your Maximized Living Doctor about the benefits of this whole food nutrients.

Research done on both elite and novice athletes shows that the benefits of low-intensity, long-duration activity are far outweighed by the benefits of high-intensity, short-duration exercise. The overall program is called surge training. This type of exercise, when applied exactly the way we will teach you, actually raises your human growth hormone (HGH), testosterone, and beta-endorphins, thus turning your body into a muscle-building, fat-burning machine. Those beta-endorphins will also give you a peace-inducing, pain-reducing high. Perhaps the best part is that the "burst" portion you will discover here only takes 12 minutes a week.

Testimonial – *Cindy Rutz, 55 years old*

Surge Training on a Replaced Hip?

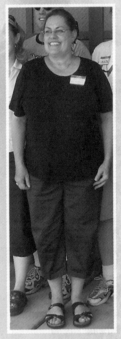

At 55 years old, I haven't felt this good about myself in years. I was not always fat. In my 30's, I wore a size 6. Then my two sons arrived, and the demands of running a business while raising a family took their toll. At some point, stress just became a way of life. Like many overweight people, I tried every diet fad there was. When the weight didn't come off fast enough, I would give up. What's worse is that I was always thinking about food!

Then along came Maximized Living. What a find! Every day I can't be thankful enough about this fantastic program. I shed 50 pounds in just six months. My husband also lost the 15 pounds he didn't need. Together we get spinal adjustments and eat the right foods. I am still amazed by how happy I am, how good I feel, and how much my husband likes my new look!

Ever since my hip replacement four or five years ago, I couldn't find an exercise I could do to help with weight loss until I found surge training! If you don't know about this, you must find out. It is easy, even if you have a disability or are 55 years old. I attribute my weight loss to the combination of diet and surge training.

Another huge bonus is that I dropped one of my medications and hope to quit the other two soon. With the help of the Maximized Living staff, I know I will accomplish this as well. This program just makes sense, if you follow their advice about eating the right foods to make your body work at its best. I'll see you all poolside on the cruise ship!

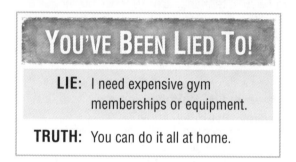

YOU'VE BEEN LIED TO!

LIE: I need expensive gym memberships or equipment.

TRUTH: You can do it all at home.

An infomercial's dream client is the person who believes fancy gadgets or exercise equipment will somehow get them miraculous results. Is this you?

Millions of dollars have been spent on late-night infomercials for exercise equipment. Indeed, most of this has been purchased because people are still too lazy to get out there and just start sweating. They have catchy headlines like: "Get ripped in five days or your money back," "Lose ten pounds in three days," or "Stay fit while you sit, or we double your money back." Unfortunately, these leave you salivating at the promise but starving for results.

The infomercial gurus are making their money betting that if you're too lazy to exercise, you're too lazy to get your money back. More than likely, you'll find most infomercial gym equipment currently operating as a towel rack or selling at a spring garage sale for 15 dollars.

There is absolutely nothing inherently wrong with home equipment, and gyms are fantastic places, but the truth is you can get the best workout of your entire life in the comfort of your own home.

The thought that you need expensive equipment is really coming from an impulsive belief in the false promises or from the mind-set that you just don't know what to do. We're offering results not promises.

Surge Training: The "New" Aerobics

Surge Training
Speaking of fat burning, you are about to learn the phenomenon called "surge training." Remember, weight loss is all about hormones. With surge training, you will release the hormones designed to burn fat and build muscle—hormones that have most likely been plummeting in your body since you were a teenager. One of these hormones is human growth hormone (HGH); the other is testosterone. It's illegal to take these drugs in sports because of their benefits. However, it's legal to produce them naturally. The key is to get your body to make them at the right levels.

Benefits of increasing HGH production are:
- Increased energy and endurance
- Reduced fat accumulation and increased lean muscle mass
- Increased bone density
- Improved libido and sexual performance
- Lower blood pressure
- Improved sleep patterns and moods

The best thing about surge training is that it only takes 12 minutes per week.

Surge training consists of short, intermittent bursts, or surges, of energy. It's similar to the concept of interval training, only done within a more limited time frame and with a strong focus on the importance of the recovery time.

The idea of the surge is to safely shock your body into responding physiologically so that you're left afterward in a more ideal metabolic state for getting toned and in better condition. After a maximum energy output, or surge, the body must respond. After a surge, it responds or adapts by altering hormones and physiology so that your body is burning fat and building muscle during and after the exercise activity.

Anyone can do surge training, and it's safe. But, as with all exercise, you should consult with your health-care professional first. However, we can say it's safe because it is built around the fact that your maximum output is what is right for you. You can go at a maximum without using heavy weights or overstraining your joints or muscles. It's a superior workout for anyone, from a beginner trying to drop pounds, to the Olympian or professional athlete trying to compete at the highest level. Here's how you get started.

First, you need to figure out your maximum heart rate. This is a vital step before you begin exercising. Here are the formulas:

MAXIMUM HEART RATE (MHR): Subtract your age from 220. The difference equals your maximum heart rate per minute.
(For example: 220–40 years old = 180 MHR)

TRAINING HEART RATE (THR): 75 to 85 percent of your MHR is your training heart rate (THR). (From the example above, 75 percent of 180 MHR = 135 beats per minute and 85 percent = 153 beats per minute. So THR = 135–153.)

Add 10 to your THR if you're an experienced athlete. As an elite athlete, you can go at or even above your MHR. (An elite athlete will see the heart rate come down quickly during recovery.)

Subtract 10 from your THR if you're a beginner or experiencing or recovering from health problems.

Now let's make this specific to you:
Fill in the blanks and do the calculations.

220 - _____ (Age) = _____ (MHR)
Training Heart Rate Range:
_____ (MHR) x .75 = _____ - _____ Lower Range
_____ (MHR) x .85 = _____ - _____ Upper Range

Experienced/elite athletes add 10
Beginners or those with health concerns subtract 10

WARNING: Stop the workout if you're not an elite athlete and your heart rate reaches 100 percent or more of your maximum heart rate, or if your heart rate jumps, or your heart rate won't go down. Consult a physician immediately.

Testimonial – *Tom Pyles, 44 years old*

In Better Shape at Age 50 Than at Age 20

As a certified fitness trainer and owner of FlexTraining, LLC, I have searched my whole life to find the secret to optimal health and fitness. I played basketball in college and began lifting weights at 30. With each new decade, I've increased my cardio endurance, strength, and overall fitness. Now at 44, I am in the best shape of my life. It may sound like a commercial, but it's true. With the help of Dr. Pellow and the Maximized Living program, I've discovered the next stage of fitness: burst or surge training.

Burst or surge training is basically doing a three-minute series of exercises of short duration but high intensity. This combination helps the body produce fat-burning hormones while challenging the heart rate and increasing overall strength. As a trainer, I have found that I can scale these exercises to anyone's fitness level, from barely mobile to highly fit. I can also adjust interval times to suit personal tastes and schedules. Best of all,

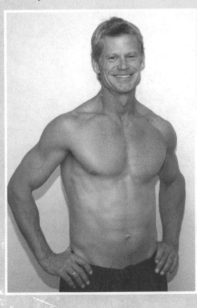

anyone can do it anywhere—no equipment or gym needed. You can select exercises you like best and/or ones you feel you need most. Surge training helps aging athletes because it puts less stress on muscles and joints than other exercises. Fewer aches and pains mean better overall fitness. I should know.

Surge training is my top secret plan to be in better shape at 50 than I was at 40, 30, or even 20! Try it. You'll be amazed.

The Surges

The reason surge training is so exciting and can be done by anyone is that in a surge set, you exercise as hard as you can (do a maximal output) for a minimum of just ten to 20 seconds and a maximum of sixty seconds (elite athletes only). Anyone can exercise or do anything for ten seconds! Because it's the maximum output for you and not someone else, surge is for everybody. It's ideal whether you're a grandma or an Olympian.

After a surge set, the secret is to recover just long enough to allow your heart rate to slow to a normal or resting heart rate, then you surge again. Recovery time is equal to the effort time. After the surge, you'll find out why even this short amount of exercise is still "aerobics." Aerobic means exercise with air, and you'll definitely be breathing more heavily and seeing your cardiovascular system getting a workout if you are surging at your maximum output.

Basic Surge Program

The forms of exercise may not be any different than the ones you may have tried in the past. It's the way you exercise that makes surge training work. Here are ten exercises you can use for surge:

1. Using a stepper alone or while curling or lifting weights from your hips to your shoulders, up over your head, and then lowering the weights to your hips again.
2. Stepping up and down on a step, without weights or while using weights as described in number 1.
3. Riding a bicycle or stationary bike.
4. Running outside or on a treadmill without weights.
*5. Running in place in a pool, with or without water weights.
6. Walking.
*7. Stepping up and down in place on the floor as fast as you can, with or without weights.
*8. Swimming laps in a pool.
9. Rollerblading.
10. Using an aerobic machine like a rower or elliptical machine.

Great for building upper and lower body muscle all at once.

Here is an example of a surge cycle:

1. 20 seconds of full-on exercise to get your heart rate quickly up close to THR.
2. 20 seconds of recovery to get heart rate back below or toward the bottom end of THR.
3. 20 seconds full on.
4. 20 seconds of recovery.
5. 20 seconds full on to complete the first cycle.

Follow the third surge/complete cycle with two minutes off. This will allow your physiology to calm or recover more completely before surging again.

6. Do two more cycles.

By repeating three cycles, you will have performed three minutes of total exercise. With recovery times during and between cycles, total elapsed time is nine minutes.

Repeat these surge workouts four times a week, and watch the results! That equals just 12 total minutes of full-on exercise, with only 36 minutes total elapsed time. That's far less than most people put into one workout, and it's your whole week!

IMPORTANT: A sixty-second surge should only be attempted by elite athletes. Once you've gone past a peak output and begin to level off, you lose some of the surge benefit and are now doing an interval. Intervals are effective, but as your body loses the shock value, they are not as effective at producing the hormonal response.

Yes, It Really Is That Simple

If you choose to run up and down on a step in your house, you would step up and down fast for 20 seconds, then rest for 20 seconds, then step again for 20 seconds, and so on. The two best things about surge training is that it takes no equipment and hardly any time.

What works better for your busy schedule—three minutes a day of exercise or 24 hours a day of being dead?

With surge training, no one can use "no time" as an excuse for not getting healthy and in the best shape of your life. Again, what works better for your busy schedule—three minutes a day of exercise or 24 hours a day of being dead?

Surge training is the most flexible, adaptable, and easy-to-fit-in exercise model with maximum benefits for your life! And it works for everyone. More advanced athletes can work this into their weekly training and/or increase the number of surges per session to radically improve their performance times. And surge times can be increased until experienced athletes are doing up to sixty-second surges.

Whether you're extremely active in everyday life or a professional athlete, you need help to reduce inflammation in joints and tissues and aid in rapid recovery following physical activity. **Max Recovery®** will help you maintain energy, recover quickly and limit potential injuries through healing nutrients such as Betaine, Coconut Water, Bromelain, Protease Enzymes and Serrapeptase.

Tips for Consistency and Guaranteed Results

- Start by circling five exercises on page 55 that you would like to do.
- Work with your local Maximized Living doctor or go to **www.maximizedliving.com** to learn more about the entire surge program. **MaxT3®** incorporates scientific principles and fierce intensity into a complete fitness system. Our 2-DVD set includes 12 workouts, with more than 80 exercise moves!

Max-Mind Moment

What Picture Have You Painted of Yourself That You Repaint Every Day?

Most people have what they are not firmly embedded in their minds. There's a saying, "Argue for your limitations and they're yours." Very true.

If you say, "I'm not a morning person," "I don't like to exercise," "I'm not very disciplined," "I just hate vegetables," "I'm lazy," "I'm a procrastinator," "I'm depressed," "I'm fat," "I'm old," or "I'm sick," then you're absolutely right!

However, if you say, "I'm a 'go-to-bed-on-time-and-get-up-ready-to-rock-and-roll-at-6:00-a.m.' kind of person," "I love the feeling I get from completing a workout," "I've found several vegetable recipes I love so much I could eat them every day," or "I'm getting fitter, younger, and healthier by the day," then you're absolutely right!

What you need is to exchange your old, lousy, self-loathing, limiting beliefs for ones that actually are moving you toward the person you dream to be, the person you were created to be, and the person you really are.

During the Lose Ten Pounds Fast phase, put your new beliefs on note cards. Also, put your big why in a place you'll clearly see several times a day. It may all seem impossible now, like we're being unrealistic, or like we're suggesting you simply start looking at the world through rose-colored glasses. First of all, what do you have to lose? Secondly, you have one body and one life to live, so why spend it boxed in by limitations when you can spend it focused on abundant possibilities? Thinking about what you're not is not a good strategy for a happy, healthy life, where you are a blessing to the people around you. Focus on what you really are and what you can become.

> Focus on what you really are and what you can become.

Examples of What Your New Beliefs Should Look Like
- Every day, my body is changing from a fat-building, muscle-burning machine to a fat-burning, muscle-building machine.

- Every day, I enjoy my new lifestyle more and more. It gives me the energy, health, and body I've always dreamed of. It's easy, not hard, to stay with this the rest of my very long life.

- As I apply the two secrets daily, they become my secret weapons for dropping ten pounds in two weeks!

Examples of What Your Big Why Should Look Like
- I want to be at my children's weddings and play catch with my grandkids.

- My husband and I plan to retire and still fulfill a purpose and take long walks down the beach.

- I want to create healthy cells for my future and not cancerous ones, as did my [mom, dad, sister, etc.]

- I am the role model for my family. If my lifestyle is great, theirs will be great.

- I want to look in the mirror and say, "You look hot naked!"

Remember, your maximized mind is your secret weapon, so write down these new beliefs on flash cards or somewhere you can easily access them and see them every day. Read them three times in the morning and three times before bed every day for 30 days. Continue daily until you have a brand new mind-set.

Also, print your big why or whys in a large font on a piece of paper. You can even color it and add pictures to make it as vivid and real as possible. Put the paper where you will see it multiple times per day.

Follow these instructions to totally reprogram the way you think and therefore the way you act, look, and feel.

CHAPTER 7

Step Four Toward the Cruise Ship
Stop Poisoning Your Family!

---

*"If you don't want it bad enough to risk losing it,
you don't want it bad enough."[1]*

—*Tom Krause*

HOW MANY PRESCRIPTION DRUGS DO you take each year? Would it surprise you to know that nearly four billion prescription drugs are ingested in the United States annually, and that more than 70,000 chemicals are used commercially? Additionally, more than 3,000 chemicals are added to our food supply, and over 10,000 are used in food processing, preserving, and storage. That's literally tons and tons of chemicals! It's also a lot of toxicity that finds its way, accidentally and on purpose, into our bodies every day. We are being poisoned—and we are giving the poison to ourselves.

Toxicity in the United States—and moving abroad as other countries adopt America's health-care model—has reached catastrophic levels. Over the past century, we have grown accustomed to the growing number of heart attacks and cancer cases. Today, we can also add to the list increases in many other diseases.

In 1970, only four in 10,000 children developed autism,[2] a brain and immune system disorder that usually develops between birth and age six. In February 2007, the Centers for Disease Control (CDC) published an analysis of 2002 data that revealed that one in 94 to one in 303 American children developed autism by age eight.[3] That's a national average of one child in every 150 or more suffering from Autism Spectrum Disorders (ASD).[4]

That's not all. One in three adults develops autoimmune diseases like multiple sclerosis, rheumatoid arthritis, and lupus, a disability in which the body's immune system starts to attack itself. In fact, America has more degenerative diseases like heart disease, cancer, arthritis, diabetes, and Alzheimer's than any other country in the world.

Even more puzzling to doctors are the numbers of people suffering from mysterious illnesses such as chronic fatigue syndrome and fibromyalgia. Add the increasing presence of diseases and disorders like attention deficit disorder and attention deficit hyperactivity disorder (in both children and adults), asthma (which has increased in children more than 10 times in the last decade), acid reflux, thyroid failure, Parkinson's, and others, and we have to ask ourselves, "What is going on, and how can we stop the madness?"

We Can Choose to Stop Poisoning Ourselves

Today, your family's ability to remain healthy, avoid suffering, and prevent disease requires looking at not one, but all Five Essentials of Maximized Living. Essential 5 requires you to acknowledge the absolute constant invasion of toxic substances into your body and the poisons that are building up as a result.

How do you know if you are toxic?

Here are some common symptoms of toxicity:

- Anxiety
- Depression
- Fatigue
- Eyelid, face, or muscle twitching
- Digestive issues
- Dizziness
- Irritability
- Muscle and joint pain
- Sensitivity to sound
- Inability to concentrate ("brain fog")
- Hormone deregulation
- Cold hands and feet
- Tinnitus (ringing in the ears)
- Sleep problems
- Overweight and weight-loss resistant

Medication—the Number-One Cause of Toxicity

Healthy lifestyles are the biggest threat to the growth and expansion of the drug industry. A recent Forbes magazine cover article, "Pharma's New Enemy: Clean Living," thoroughly addressed this subject from the position of the consumer as well as the investor. Consider the following perspective from the article: "Do you really need all those prescription and over the counter pills you are popping? Maybe not. There's a backlash building against the cost, risk and side effects of medication, and it's bad news for the pharmaceutical industry."[5]

The message was driven home even more powerfully when the article noted: "The results of pill dependence are insidious and devastating: billions of dollars in ever-higher drug costs; millions of people enduring sometimes highly toxic side-effects; and close to 2 million cases each year of drug complications that result in 180,000 deaths or life-threatening illnesses in the elderly."[6]

As the article notes, "Every few years the ultimate medical catastrophe: a miracle cure that turns out to be toxic."[7] (Think Vioxx, Avandia, hormone-replacement therapy, Paxil, and the like.) Every drug is a toxin!

It used to be that an apple a day would keep the doctor away. The recommendation now is an aspirin a day. It turns out, however, that an aspirin a day for at least five years increases a woman's chance of developing breast cancer by 80 percent.[8] Seems like a good idea to take your chances with the apple.

If you get breast cancer, chances are that the drugs prescribed will cause more harm than good. Many women have been prescribed Tamoxifen. Research now shows that taking Tamoxifen increases the chance of incidence and death from uterine cancer.[9]

Even something as seemingly harmless as over-the-counter children's cough medicine can be deadly. A cough rarely kills a child, but cough medicine and cough syrup just might. The CDC recently released a warning to parents after more than 1,500 infants and toddlers wound up in emergency rooms and three children died because of reactions to overdoses of pediatric cold medicines. Behind the scenes, one doctor admitted, "Fluids and patience are the best treatment."[10]

The most common prescription drugs sold in the U.S. today, and possibly the most toxic to your system, are antidepressant medications. Possible side effects include suicide, aggressive behavior, nausea, insomnia, anxiety, restlessness, decreased sex drive, dizziness, weight gain or loss, tremors, sweating, sleepiness, fatigue, dry mouth, diarrhea, constipation, headaches, and on and on. Clearly, the issues of toxicity are severe with this type of drug.

> The most common prescription drugs sold in the U.S. today, and possibly the most toxic to your system, are antidepressant medications.

If you look at the top 20 best-selling drugs in the U.S., you will be amazed by two things: the sheer dollars spent and what they are prescribed for. The top drugs sold are for pain, heart disease, heartburn, and many other conditions that could easily be prevented by applying what you've learned in this book.

As you've heard in the past, there is no free lunch. That is the case with medication. Even if the drug makes the symptom go away, you will pay the price on the back-end with the side effects of toxicity; side effects that sooner or later tend to turn out worse than the condition the drug was prescribed for in the first place. You want to know what really puts a whole lot of people in the nursing home instead of in a suite on a cruise ship? It's often the pills they're taking or have been taking for years.

Testimonial — *Gralyn Farris, 53 years old*

Just Say No

I worked as a pharmaceutical tech for 10 years. What I noticed during that time about the use of drugs and their side effects really bothered me. I watched doctors prescribe drugs, supposedly to help people, without ever actually tackling the underlying problem. They would give patients drugs as a crutch to help them get through some crisis, but then leave them on the drugs with no attempt to really improve their health. Sometimes, they had to give them more drugs to counteract the side effects of the first drugs!

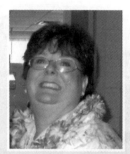

I was trapped in that vicious circle too. For 10 years or more, I was sad, anxious, stressed, and my body hurt in odd ways that no one could diagnose. So naturally, they suggested antidepressants and antianxiety pills, as well as meds for high blood pressure, hormones, and pain. It was far too easy to ask for more pills, because doctors always wanted to help you feel better but not actually get better. The drugs kept me stuck, surviving, but not feeling well. It's hard to admit that exercise, nutrition, detox, and chiropractic adjustments are the answer for change. The problem is, the drugs keep you from change. I wonder how many of us are out there living a half-life and thinking, "Is this all there is?"

Maximized Living has taught me to respect my body and to embrace change. I learned to eat right, exercise, and get the toxins out of my body. That, plus adjustments, allowed my body to heal itself. Now, my body is a drug-free zone, where I experience life the way it is—happy, sad, easy, or hard—without chemical interference. I trust my body to show me the way. My health is back in my own hands and I feel great, thanks to Maximized Living. Maximized Living stands for change and a choice! I choose to be drug-free, I choose to feel good, and I choose what I put in my body! I thank Maximized Living for giving me the power to say no to drugs.

You can't eliminate all toxins, but you can trust your body to do what it was created to do. When it is working at its optimum level—healing and functioning normally—your body is made to process and remove a certain amount of poison, but not the amounts in "modern" Western living.

It's critical for you to become aware of the "Toxic Top Five" and eliminate them as much as possible in order to live the principle of essential 5 of Maximized Living.

The Toxic Top Five

1. Medications

If you are taking medications for chronic conditions, do what Gralyn did. Start making lifestyle changes and let your doctor know what you are doing. Ask for his or her help to reduce the medications.

2. Household products

Household cleaners

Every product with a Caution, Warning, or Danger label may add deadly chemicals to your body through either your mouth, your skin, or by inhaling fumes. Many add up over time and can be stored in the liver or fat cells. Children, in particular, are at high risk. Some of the most potent toxins are hidden in your cabinets. They are dishwashing detergents, oven cleaners, laundry detergent, floor and furniture polishes, air fresheners, hard-surface cleaners (especially kitchen cleaners), antibacterial cleaners and soaps, dry cleaning, carpet and upholstery cleaners, and toilet bowl cleaners.

What to Watch Out For

According to www.organicconsumers.org: When consumers buy commercial cleaning products, we expect them to do one thing: clean! We use a wide array of scents, soaps, detergents, bleaching agents, softeners, scourers, polishes, and specialized cleaners for bathrooms, glass, drains, and ovens to keep our homes sparkling and sweet-smelling. But, while the chemicals in cleaners, foam, bleach, and disinfectants do make our dishes, bathtubs, and countertops gleaming and germ-free, many also contribute to indoor air pollution, are poisonous if ingested, and can be harmful if inhaled or touched. In fact, some cleaners are among the most toxic products found in the home. In 2000, cleaning products were responsible for nearly 10 percent of all toxic exposures reported to U.S. Poison Control Centers, accounting for 206,636 calls. Of these, 120,434 exposures involved children under six, who can swallow or spill cleaners stored or left open inside the home.

Cleaning ingredients vary in the type of health hazard they pose. Some cause acute, or immediate, hazards such as skin or respiratory irritation, watery eyes, or chemical burns, while others are associated with chronic, or long-term effects, such as cancer.[11]

Personal care products
These toxins are hiding in your bathroom. They are in your shower and by your sink. Changing the personal care products that you use can have an incredibly positive effect on your family's health. Read the labels on your soap, conditioner, shampoo, and toothpaste.

What to Watch Out For

- **Diethanolamine (DEA)** is found in over six hundred home and personal care products such as soaps, lotions, cosmetics, bubble baths, and laundry and dishwashing detergents. In 1997, the U.S. Department of Health and Human Services National Toxicity Program found that when DEA was applied to the skin of rats, it resulted in clear evidence of carcinogenic (cancerous) activity.[12]

- **Propylene glycol** is a substance used as a powerful solvent in antifreeze solutions and hydraulic fluids. Ironically enough, it is also found in childhood vaccinations, cosmetics, toothpastes, shampoos, deodorants, lotions, and even processed foods (including pet foods). Like DEA, propylene glycol has been shown in studies to be absorbed through the skin and cause many problems, such as kidney damage, liver abnormalities, skin cell growth inhibition, damaged cell membranes, rashes, respiratory damage, immune system deficiency, and central nervous system depression.[13]

- **Sodium lauryl sulfate (SLS)** is perhaps the most common of the three chemicals and by no means any less toxic. SLS is used as a surfactant to break down the surface tension of water. This degreaser is used in practically every soap, shampoo, and toothpaste on the market today. SLS has been used in studies to induce mutation in bacteria and to irritate skin. It has also been shown to enter the heart, liver, lungs, and brain from skin contact and has been proven to maintain residual levels once inside these organs.[14]

Solution: Use natural products that do not contain these chemicals. They are available online and at most health food stores.

3. Teflon cookware
What to Watch Out For

Teflon contains Perfluorooctanoic Acid (PFOA), which has been shown to cause tumors in rats, along with "serious changes in the weight of various organs, including the brain, prostate, liver, thymus, and kidneys, along with damage to the pituitary at all doses in female rat offspring," according the Environmental Working Group. The pituitary is important because it secretes hormones that regulate growth, reproduction, and many metabolic processes. Change in pituitary size is associated with toxicity. The EPA unanimously voted that PFOA should be considered a likely carcinogen in humans and has called for a ban by 2015.

An article in the Washington Post sums up why you want to get rid of your Teflon pans:

"Teflon Chemicals Are a Threat to Health"

Dupont recently defended its position about partially complying with federal reporting guidelines on the health risks of a key ingredient found in Teflon.

The chemical giant has been criticized on many sides for its decision not to release all the information it compiled on Perfluorooctanoic Acid (PFOA), a soap-like ingredient used in making nonstick surfaces and materials. As a result, EPA has sought fines up to $300 million, arguing the company failed to inform the government and public about PFOA.

The concerns:

DuPont concealed its own 1981 research showing traces of the chemical in a pregnant worker's unborn child.

10 years later, the company failed to report evidence that the chemical had contaminated the water supply of 12,000 people.

The son of a DuPont factory worker, who was born with only one nostril and other facial defects (he has had 30 operations), is one of eight families suing the company over PFOA. Although the man recently married, he and his spouse have opted not to have children, in case they inherit his condition....A senior scientist at the Environmental Working Group pointed out that PFOA, like other fluorochemicals, is in people everywhere, never breaks down in the environment, and is toxic at or near levels found in humans.

Another health issue, "Teflon flu" causes aches and pains when nonstick pans are overheated, although a DuPont spokesperson said the physical problems are temporary and pass quickly. Yet birds, particularly small ones like finches and cockatiels, can die in short order from those kitchen fumes.[15]

– Washington Post, August 13, 2004

Solution: If it is going to be banned, why would you keep letting it poison your family? Go to your cabinets, pull out anything that is nonstick and throw it away now! Buy stainless steel cookware. Use Extra Virgin Olive Oil at low to moderate heats and Coconut Oil at high heats to reduce sticking.

4. Tap water
What to Watch Out For

Tap water is full of Chlorine, heavy metals, contaminants, and other toxins. Chlorine is a big one. If it is strong enough to kill bacteria and other dangerous stuff in our water, do you really think it's a good idea to drink it? It doesn't end at Chlorine, though. Many studies have found prescription drugs, including beta-blockers, estrogen, antidepressants, and pain killers in tap water. Tap water also contains heavy metals and other horrendous things that make their way into your house. It's up to you whether they make it into your body.

A 2006 article in the International Journal of Cancer had this to say about tap water: "Six recent studies, examining a combined total of almost 8,000 people, have indicated that higher consumption of tap water can increase the risk of bladder cancer in men. Men who drank more than two liters of tap water a day ran a 50 percent higher risk of bladder cancer than those who drank half a liter or less. Both straight tap water and tap water from other sources, such as coffee, were examined in the study. Other beverages were not found to have the same associated risks."[16]

So bottled water must be the answer, right? Wrong! An Environmental Working Group (EWG) investigation of almost 200 popular bottled water brands found that less than two percent disclosed the water's source, how the water has been purified, and what chemical pollutants each bottle of water may contain.[17] So, you don't know where it's coming from or what's still in it.

The average American uses 170 plastic water bottles in one year, totaling 50 billion plastic bottles a year. In fact, Americans spend more than 15 billion dollars on bottled water every single year! [18]

Solution: Get a water filter. There are plenty of good filters out there, but we recommend reverse osmosis filters. A four-stage reverse osmosis filter removes the impurities from water and will save you hundreds of dollars per year compared to buying water. Also, when you drink the water, drink it out of a water bottle that is not plastic. Plastics contain Phthalates. Also, store your food in glass containers instead of plastic. Stainless steel water bottles are best for repeat use.

5. Mold and Biotoxins

Mold has certainly made its way into people's homes as well as the headlines recently. Many people still don't fully understand the health hazards of fungal exposure. The term toxic mold is somewhat misleading as it exudes an idea that certain molds are toxic, when actually certain types of molds produce something called Mycotoxins. Airborne Mycotoxins can definitely destroy one's health. Sometimes, people are unaware that they are breathing mold spores and Mycotoxins until they are very sick. Certain people have a minor allergic reactions to the some molds, However, if they have been exposed to the dangerous molds they could suffer from a myriad of serious symptoms and illnesses such as chronic bronchitis, learning disabilities, mental deficiencies, heart problems, cancer, multiple sclerosis, chronic fatigue, lupus, fibromyalgia, rheumatoid arthritis, multiple chemical sensitivity, bleeding lungs and much more.

Unfortunately, the government has failed to establish guidelines that determine unhealthful amounts of poor indoor air quality standards, making it impossible for thousands of sick people to obtain help. This is the main reason why so many people are confused about the damage mold can cause. As most know, many molds can cause allergens that can affect some of the population, but some molds can also cause toxins, which can affect everyone, depending on the length of exposure. Approximately 25 million Americans suffer from allergic reactions to molds yet most of them don't even realize that when they're sneezing and sniffling the cause could be from fungi. The molds that produce airborne toxins that can cause serious symptoms, such as breathing difficulties, memory and hearing loss, dizziness, flu-like symptoms, and acid reflux and weakened immune systems. Eyesight, memory, coordination/balance, and hearing can also be affected.

Molds can be found wherever there is moisture and oxygen. Molds grow in our homes in moist warm areas like damp basements, closets, and bathrooms, even after the moisture has dried up. Also, molds can grow in places where fresh food is stored, refrigerator drip trays, house plants, humidifiers, garbage pails, mattresses, upholstered furniture, or foam rubber pillows. The worst place that molds can grow, however, is inside wall cavities and flooring of our homes, wherever there may be cellulose materials they can feed on, such as wood and ceiling tiles.

Testimonial – *Jerry Little, 63 years old*
Whispers of Truth

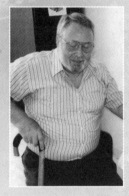

I wanted to take the time and reflect on where I am. Although I am not where I want to be, I believe God is smiling because I finally heard His whispers telling me what to do — and that was Maximized Living! Even from the beginning of care in February, I began to feel subtle improvements, but they were slower than my dreams had hoped for. Then it happened. In a little more than 30 days, I have gone from being a legal prescription drug addict with multiple major health problems, to the best I have felt in

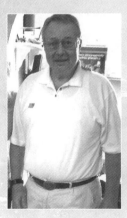

15 years. This includes, but is not limited to, a much-improved quality of life and more stamina than I had previously dreamed would occur. The food detox diet and supplemental detox program has been a complete miracle! Did I mention that I am 63 years old years old and have been medically and legally classified as totally and permanently disabled by highly trained medical specialists? I cannot thank Maximized Living enough, as they have changed my life!

What to Do About It

In the 28 day challenge you will eliminate the Toxic Top 5 to reduce your toxic burden. Even with that, however, toxins are unavoidable in the times we are living. That's why it is important to clear out your detoxification pathways to neutralize and clean out the junk that you are exposed to on a daily basis. The best way to do that is **Daily Detox®**.

Exposure to everyday toxins can affect you down to the cellular level. Toxicity can cause fatigue, inflammation, weight gain, depression, and has been linked to cancer. **Daily Detox®** is a whole food formula unlike any other detox formula because it utilizes a two fold approach to cleanse your system. First, it cleanses with traditional organ system detoxifiers like Chorella, Milk Thistle, Spirulina and Probiotics. Then it protects your cells against free radical damage with intracellular antioxidants like Glutathione, Catalase and Superoxide. Second, **Daily Detox®** is unique in that it has specific nutrients to shuttle toxins out of your body. The special formulation of activated charcoal and Magnesium effectively bind to toxins, helping your body safely eliminate them.

Inevitably, toxins that surround you every day in foods, medications, beverages and even in the air migrate into your bloodstream. Now the body has to work on a never ending basis to detoxify chemicals, parasites and heavy metals. You can't afford to let these chemicals stay in your bloodstream causing disease and hardship down the line!

CHAPTER 8

Step Five Toward the Cruise Ship
Turn Your Power On!

"My people perish for lack of knowledge."

—*Hosea* 4:6

Testimonial – *Carol Montayne, 51 years old*

A Chiropractic E-mail of Hope

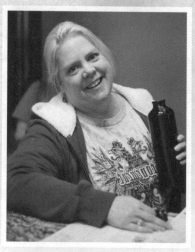

Sorry this took so long. It's been a rough day. So, I can come more than three times a week? How can we work that out? I feel pretty anxious over all this and somewhat scared, but at the same time, I'm really excited. This is a chance for my life to be completely changed. To have hope is a brand new feeling. I just didn't know where to turn anymore. Daryl is supporting me fully, and he's already said he too will do whatever it takes.

I have been prescribed a long list of medications that include:

- Trexall—10 mg, two times a week
- Mobic—7.5 mg, two times a day
- Baclofen—20 mg, three times a day
- Naproxen Sodium—550 mg, two times a day
- Oxycodone/APAP—325 mg, daily
- Endocet—two pills, every six hours as needed
- Prednisone—10 mg, every other day
- Neurontin—up to 1800 mg, daily or as needed for pain relief
- Phillips' Milk of Magnesia as needed
- Fleet Enema as needed
- Dulcolax as needed
- Ditropan—5 mg, three times a day
- Hiprex—1 g, two times a day
- Cyclobnzaprine/Flexeril—10 mg, three times a day
- Fentanyl transdermal duragesic 75 (three-day patch)
- Tamadol—100 mg, every four to six hours as needed
- Soma—350 mg, two times a day
- Trazodone—50 mg, one a day
- Acetaminophen, two times a day
- Skelaxin—800mg, two pills
- Ativan—1 mg, three times a day
- Prozac—60 mg, one time a day
- Valium—10 mg, three times a day
- Avapro—150 mg, one time a day
- Excedrin Migraine—three pills every four hours as needed
- Ibuprofen—800 mg, four times a day

These are all on the shelf. I can take all of them at times, but I've been told I can pretty much pick and choose depending on how I feel with them since most of them deal with pain or are anxiety related. I don't like how they make me feel because I feel like a zombie all of the time and have a constant hangover feeling. All I want to do is sleep when I'm on this stuff. It's a no-win situation. I don't understand how these doctors can just keep prescribing one thing on top of another with no concern about the side effects. It seems to me that there must be something out there in nature that is natural that could help rather than all these man-made chemicals, but my brain is so fogged. Then comes the difficulty that there are tons of information from so many sources. Who do you trust? The decision has been made.

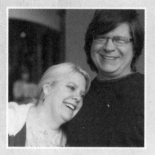

I'm getting off all this junk somehow. You are my doctor now. You have the training, so I'm going to trust you to get me to the point where I can think clearly once again and let you show and teach me the right resources. I am a mess—really I am—and I can't go on this way or I'll be dead, one way or another. I am so desperate. I realize that it's probably going to be rough in the beginning because I'm dependent. But I will do anything to be whole again. This life has no meaning like this....

Carol's e-mail after starting chiropractic and the Five Essentials:

I have my life back in such a short time—no meds, no cane, and losing weight and inches. After years of suffering with Rheumatoid Arthritis, Multiple Sclerosis, and Fibromyalgia, I am alive again. The real test for me was what would happen when the weather changed and we'd get rain. That used to put me to bed. I sailed right through it all this past week. I sleep at night, when I never could before without sleeping meds. My blood pressure is now normal, when before I was taking meds for that, too. I have energy. I don't know that I have ever felt so good. I was one very sick girl! So what was it that made the amazing difference? Everything. Not just one aspect of this Maximized Living program, but all of it combined. I don't want the old lifestyle back; it isn't worth it! I can only imagine three to six months from now! I have the goal now, and the prize is set before me.... People are amazed. I spent a good ten minutes just sharing with folks today at the Vitamin Shoppe. Even the manager asked about how things changed so fast! I used to be so afraid of the holiday season, but I'm actually excited about overcoming this time! All I know is this: it works.

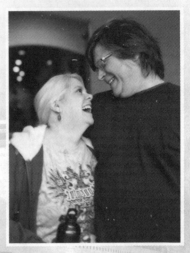

We made wrong choices. Thank you for teaching me the right ways. You are a blessing and an answer to a prayer! If you ever want to share with others what has happened, go ahead.

I never did go get that handicapped placard. I don't need it!

People perish for lack of knowledge, and in Carol's case, she didn't realize what she didn't know. However, it doesn't take a rocket scientist to realize that if you don't take care of something, eventually it's only a matter of time before it breaks down. You brush your teeth to prevent cavities, you put oil in your car to prevent the engine from falling out, and you change the furnace filter to prevent a temperature meltdown. You don't wait until your teeth are rotting, the engine starts smoking, or your A/C or heater blows up before you look into taking care of them, do you?

Your spine is the exact same way. If all you do is use and abuse it but don't provide proper care and maintenance, it's going to quite literally rot, break down, or blow up on you. As crazy as it seems, people do wait for smoke to start coming out of their spine before they do something about it. If you don't believe it, just look at the nearly 350,000 back surgeries performed every year. You should have been maintaining your spine from birth. So if you're a little late in giving your spine the attention it needs, that's OK. While ten years ago is always the best time to have started taking care of yourself, the second best time is right now. Let's get started with the most common myth I always hear about spinal care.

> You should have been maintaining your spine from birth.

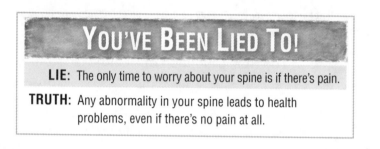

YOU'VE BEEN LIED TO!

LIE: The only time to worry about your spine is if there's pain.

TRUTH: Any abnormality in your spine leads to health problems, even if there's no pain at all.

Pain is always the last symptom to appear, long after the damage is done. The condition of your spine is crucial to the health of your organs. The nerves control the organs and, the truth is, if there is interference in those nerves, it will produce other health-related disorders. That's why Essential 2, "Maximized Nerve Supply," is not a recommendation but a mandatory essential.

The most famous example of the importance of your spinal cord is actor Christopher Reeve, who you probably know as "Superman." He fell off a horse and pushed a spinal bone from his upper neck into his lower brain, upper spinal cord area. You could measure the amount of damage in his spine with the tip of your pinkie. Yet, that's all it took for his organs to shut down. The only reason he didn't die right away is because he had machines and surgeries to keep him alive. Even though the problem was at the top of his body, they had to push on his stomach to make him go to the bathroom.

Because the power from Mr. Reeve's brain and spinal cord was blocked, nothing worked normally, and the areas most directly affected didn't work at all. The absence of nerve flow simply causes organs to shut down. On the other hand, 100 percent nerve flow gives 100 percent life to the organs.

> The fasted way to end up in the nursing home is to base your health on how you feel.

It's really that simple. If you cut the nerve that goes to your heart, what happens? It stops. If you block the nerves that go to your heart, what happens to your heart? It malfunctions. That malfunction could mean high blood pressure, irregular heartbeat, or the worst symptom of all, you feel nothing wrong until you have a heart attack that kills you on your way out to the mailbox.

Remember, the fastest way to end up in the nursing home is to base your health on how you feel. You can only base your health on how you function.

The Real Definition of Health

Every day, thousands die of heart attacks with no previous warnings, or are diagnosed with cancer even though there are no symptoms. The real definition of health, then, is when all of the cells of the body are functioning and healing at 100 percent, not simply when someone has no disease, no illness, and no pain.

Truth be told, by the time other diagnostic tests for cancer, heart disease, diabetes, Alzheimer's, and so on ever detects the illness, it's too late. You already have the condition and, at best, are now fighting for your life.

How important do you think it is for you and your family to know how well your bodies are functioning and healing?

The fact is that your spine controls all of your functions and all of the healing in your body. Therefore, if you are experiencing any symptoms like headaches, high blood pressure, digestive problems, thyroid issues, or immune system or menstrual problems, it can be coming from nerves that are not functioning.

> The real definition of health then is when all of the cells of the body are functioning and healing at 100 percent, not simply when someone has no disease, no illness, and no pain.

Look at the "Chart of the Effects of Spinal Damage" on the next page to determine which nerves could be involved with your condition.

You have to think of it this way: your spinal cord sits inside of your spinal column. Your spinal cord controls every single function in your body. If your spine goes down the tubes, your future goes with it—no cruise ship.

We see patients like this every day whose spines are literally decaying, leaving them on multiple medications, in a wheelchair, or staring at the ceiling of a nursing home. You can take out a tooth that is rotting and decaying, but you can't take out a vertebra that is rotting and decaying. You have to live with what you have.

Most of these people tell us that they would have taken care of their spines if they would have known better. Well, now you know, so you can choose to live happily or miserably—cruise ship or nursing home. The choice is yours.

Why You Are Sick: Chart of the Effects of Spinal Damage

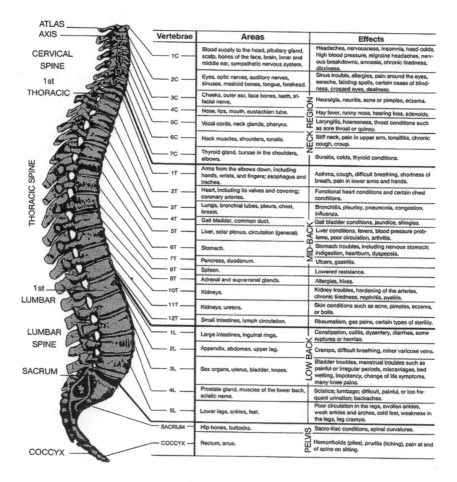

Vertebrae	Areas	Effects
1C	Blood supply to the head, pituitary gland, scalp, bones of the face, brain, inner and middle ear, sympathetic nervous system.	Headaches, nervousness, insomnia, head colds, high blood pressure, migraine headaches, nervous breakdowns, amnesia, chronic tiredness, dizziness.
2C	Eyes, optic nerves, auditory nerves, sinuses, mastoid bones, tongue, forehead.	Sinus trouble, allergies, pain around the eyes, earache, fainting spells, certain cases of blindness, crossed eyes, deafness.
3C	Cheeks, outer ear, face bones, teeth, trifacial nerve.	Neuralgia, neuritis, acne or pimples, eczema.
4C	Nose, lips, mouth, eustachian tube.	Hay fever, runny nose, hearing loss, adenoids.
5C	Vocal cords, neck glands, pharynx.	Laryngitis, hoarseness, throat conditions such as sore throat or quinsy.
6C	Neck muscles, shoulders, tonsils.	Stiff neck, pain in upper arm, tonsillitis, chronic cough, croup.
7C	Thyroid gland, bursae in the shoulders, elbows.	Bursitis, colds, thyroid conditions.
1T	Arms from the elbows down, including hands, wrists, and fingers; esophagus and trachea.	Asthma, cough, difficult breathing, shortness of breath, pain in lower arms and hands.
2T	Heart, including its valves and covering; coronary arteries.	Functional heart conditions and certain chest conditions.
3T	Lungs, bronchial tubes, pleura, chest, breast.	Bronchitis, pleurisy, pneumonia, congestion, influenza.
4T	Gall bladder, common duct.	Gall bladder conditions, jaundice, shingles.
5T	Liver, solar plexus, circulation (general).	Liver conditions, fevers, blood pressure problems, poor circulation, arthritis.
6T	Stomach.	Stomach troubles, including nervous stomach; indigestion, heartburn, dyspepsia.
7T	Pancreas, duodenum.	Ulcers, gastritis.
8T	Spleen.	Lowered resistance.
9T	Adrenal and supra-renal glands.	Allergies, hives.
10T	Kidneys.	Kidney troubles, hardening of the arteries, chronic tiredness, nephritis, pyelitis.
11T	Kidneys, ureters.	Skin conditions such as acne, pimples, eczema, or boils.
12T	Small intestines, lymph circulation.	Rheumatism, gas pains, certain types of sterility.
1L	Large intestines, inguinal rings.	Constipation, colitis, dysentery, diarrhea, some ruptures or hernias.
2L	Appendix, abdomen, upper leg.	Cramps, difficult breathing, minor varicose veins.
3L	Sex organs, uterus, bladder, knees.	Bladder troubles, menstrual troubles such as painful or irregular periods, miscarriages, bed wetting, impotency, change of life symptoms, many knee pains.
4L	Prostate gland, muscles of the lower back, sciatic nerve.	Sciatica; lumbago; difficult, painful, or too frequent urination; backaches.
5L	Lower legs, ankles, feet.	Poor circulation in the legs, swollen ankles, weak ankles and arches, cold feet, weakness in the legs, leg cramps.
SACRUM	Hip bones, buttocks.	Sacro-iliac conditions, spinal curvatures.
COCCYX	Rectum, anus.	Hemorrhoids (piles), pruritis (itching), pain at end of spine on sitting.

How Chiropractic Saved This Doctor's Life

By Dr. Chris Pellow

It was an 18 year-old's dream to spend the day on a golf course getting a great tan and relaxing while cutting lush green fairways in the warm sun. My work was enjoyable and fun, but the best part was being finished by 2:30 p.m. and having the entire summer to relax and golf all day. But after just a month on the job, I was waking up with lower back pain. At first, the pain wasn't that bad, but soon it turned into excruciating pain that radiated into the backs of my legs.

The pain was intense and felt like someone was sticking a hot knife in my back. It affected me so much that I had to sit down every half hour just to relieve the pressure. I couldn't understand what was wrong! I was only eighteen years old. I asked myself how this could be happening to me. What would my future look like if the pain didn't resolve itself, and what about my hopes and dreams?

Needless to say, I was scared. Before I knew it, I was taking a ton of toxic medications and didn't know what to do. My mother had taken me to every specialist you could think of. Finally, someone recommended that we go see a chiropractor. Funny thing is that back then I had never even heard the word chiropractor and didn't know how much it would change my life forever. After suffering with severe debilitating lower back pain for four months, I was completely pain free in only two weeks! I felt like I had my life back and couldn't believe how amazing I felt. I had actually forgotten what it felt like to feel good again. Interestingly enough, patients now tell me that all the time when they have had the same amazing results!

The real miracle was yet to come though, and I want to tell you what inspired this small town kid to travel half way across the country to go to chiropractic school in Marietta, GA. As my back pain started to go away, I also noticed that all the migraine headaches, allergy, and asthma problems didn't seem to be bothering me anymore. In fact, I never had another migraine, watery eye, stuffy nose, or asthma attack again!

That's when I learned the single most important principle of my entire life: the body doesn't need any help in healing; it just doesn't need any interference! This principle is what inspired me to become a chiropractor, write this book, and help others see the potential they have to heal without drugs or surgery. The interference was taken off of my nervous system, and my body healed itself.

Chiropractic completely saved my life, and it will do the same for you, if you are willing to allow it!

Testimonial — *Stefanie Strawn-Gentry, 28 years old*

28 Is Too Young to Give Up!

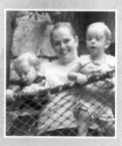

Before I met the Maximized Living team, I was really struggling. My health appeared to be on a permanent downhill slide. It started as a teen when I developed severe migraine headaches. Then at age 19 I became depressed. No wonder! Can you imagine how debilitating those headaches were? None of the drugs seemed to help. The next blow came when I developed rheumatoid arthritis at 26. I had just given birth to beautiful twin boys. The joint pain was horrible. Not only could I not lose the weight I gained in pregnancy, but also the drugs, depression, and inability to exercise caused me to pack it on. At 27 years old, I hit my max weight of 240 pounds.

My low point came in June 2008, when I was taking two types of antidepressants, along with Prednisone (a steroid), several anti-inflammatory pills, Methotrexate, and at least one Vicodin per week for my headaches. I had tried everything that medical doctors offered me, but they couldn't

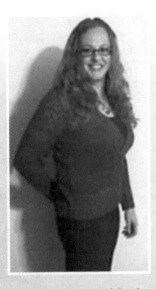

fix my problems. All those drugs were just treating my symptoms. But I still felt awful, and the weight just wouldn't come off.

The worst part was that I really needed to feel well. If you've had kids, you know that running after a toddler is hard enough. Try doubling that and doing it with 100 extra pounds and constant joint pain, migraines, and depression to boot! Without the sweet smiles on those two little faces, I don't know how I would have gotten out of bed.

I never thought about seeing a chiropractor before. In fact, I was a little bit nervous. But the chiropractor explained everything to me, and it made complete sense. I was looking for relief from my joint pain, headaches, and depression, but I had no idea that he would help me lose weight too. I started the diet program at 227 pounds, and in only eight months, I lost 54 pounds. Now, I never miss my chiropractic appointments, I follow the Advanced Eating Plan religiously, and I follow the exercise plan to a "T." Even more exciting to me is the fact that I no longer take a single medication. Not one! I don't suffer anymore from rheumatoid arthritis, depression, or migraines. I am back to the person I was made to be. Their motto was right: my body didn't need any help, just no interference. I would not be where—or who—I am today if not for the Maximized Living program.

Chiropractic Adjustments Better than
Medications for Blood Pressure?

Look at this study conducted at the University of Chicago Hypertension Center that showed that a special chiropractic adjustment can significantly lower high blood pressure: "This procedure has the effect of not one, but two blood-pressure medications given in combination," study leader George Bakris, MD, tells WebMD. "And it seems to be adverse-event free. We saw no side effects and no problems."[1]

Listen to the actual results below; they are absolutely unbelievable. There was an average 14 mm Hg greater drop in systolic blood pressure (the top number in a blood pressure count), and an average 8 mm Hg greater drop in diastolic blood pressure (the bottom blood pressure number). "When the statistician brought me the data, I actually didn't believe it. It was way too good to be true," Bakris said.[2]

The statistician responded, "I don't even believe it. But we checked for everything and there it was."

That's enough evidence right there for you to go find your nearest Maximized Living chiropractor and have your spine professionally examined, especially if you have never had a spinal examination.

There are about 72 million people in the United States age 20 and older with hypertension. This means that currently one in three adults have high blood pressure and could be benefitting from specific chiropractic adjustments.

One of the most amazing studies ever performed on chiropractic proved beyond a shadow of a doubt that the full function of the nervous system is essential for you to be healthy. This study was done at the University of Pennsylvania by Dr. Henry Winsor. He conducted an experiment based on chiropractors' claims that misalignments of the spine lead to disease. In this experiment, he dissected both human and animal cadavers to see if there was any relationship between diseased internal organs and the vertebrae and nerves that went to those organs.

Dr. Winsor dissected 75 human and 72 cat cadavers. He found a nearly 100 percent correlation between minor curvatures of the vertebrae and diseases of the internal organs.[3] If you are reading this information and already see a Maximized Living chiropractor, then congratulations. But if you have never seen a chiropractor before, then I suggest you get moving.

Testimonial – *The Renfroe Family*

NEVER GIVE UP

P Having a child with cerebral palsy is not easy. Having a special needs child with four other siblings is even more difficult.

Our daughter was born premature and there were many difficulties during her delivery. Over time it became more and more obvious that something was not right with her. She was initially diagnosed with global delays because, at eight months, she could not hold her head up, sit up, roll over or anything else. After months of physical, occupational, and speech therapy, and countless tests, she was diagnosed with cerebral

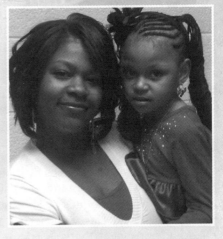

palsy by the top specialist at Children's Hospital. That was very hard to hear and even harder to accept. We have four other children that are perfectly healthy. Our daughter made slow progress over the next two years with the therapy she received. I was becoming increasingly more depressed about the situation and the outlook. The doctors gave us no hope for a better quality of life for her. They basically told us that she would be like an infant for the rest of her life. It became more and more difficult to care for her the older and bigger she got.

My sister had been inviting me to come to a Maximized Living makeover, for about three months. I was not interested because I had already been to a chiropractor and he was not much help to me and I did not want to waste my time on another one. Finally, I gave in and my husband and I went to hear a Maximized Living doctor speak. I was still not convinced, but my husband decided that we would give it a try. At our first adjustment, I was not sure what to expect but I did not expect much. When our daughter was done with her adjustment she was very happy and excited. I had never seen her respond to anything with such excitement, before. We decided that this was something we NEEDED to give a chance. When we first started, our daughter was not able to sit up without support, speak, or hold her weight on her legs. She is now able to sit like a normal child, she says words clearly and understandably, and she can stand on her legs and is in the process of learning how to walk. These are things that the doctors said she would never do. Our family has benefited in ways we could not have foreseen. Our other children are doing and feeling better than they ever have. I feel like I have a new lease on life, thanks to the results I have seen in my own body, we have been being adjusted for seven months now and can't believe the results.

Thanks to the Maximized Living doctors the power inside of her body has been unlocked and the healing virtue is flowing through her. She has amazed the therapists that have been with her for the past three and a half years. They never expected to see such progress from her and definitely not this quickly. I thank God for sending us to the Maximized Living clinic and for restoring my faith in her healing.

Maximized Nerve Supply

The body can go days without water, weeks without food, and minutes without oxygen, but it cannot last even a second without the power provided through the nervous system.

There is a physical condition called Vertebral Subluxation that commonly occurs as a result of the regular physical, mental, and chemical stress that people go through in varying levels every day.

A vertebral subluxation is any minor or major misalignment of a vertebra or several vertebrae (Global Subluxation). These misalignments, some so small that they have to be measured with an instrument, invade spinal cord space, put pressure on the spinal cord, compress nerves, and/or push soft tissue out of the way and into delicate neurological tissue.[4]

Subluxations at the top of the spine, the area where Christopher Reeve was injured, also cause pressure or damage to the brain stem— spinal cord intersection—the area of the nervous system responsible for breathing, heart rate, and vital automatic functions. (This was the area corrected in the University of Chicago blood pressure study that lowered blood pressure better than two medications combined.)

Determining How Well Your Spine Is Positioned
Determines Cruise Ship or Nursing Home

The only way to evaluate the level of nerve supply your organs are getting is by evaluating the spine. The two primary methods for evaluating proper alignment and position of the spine are X-rays and posture.

X-ray

Let's teach you how to read an X-ray. The most accurate method for measuring healthy nerve supply is to see it with the use of X-rays. When looking at the front-view X-ray, the spinal should be straight. Curvatures to the side, called Scoliosis, are such an important health concern that all children in the U.S. are checked for it in school.

The side-view X-ray must reveal three well-placed arcs. The most important arc is in the neck (cervical spine). This cervical arc is known as the Arc of Life, because life impulses travel directly from the brain down this arc, bringing life to all of the organs of the body.

You can't concoct a study that would show that losing your Arc of Life doesn't cause damage to the spinal cord, nerves, and other soft tissues. A groundbreaking study published in the medical journal Spine shows the vital need for normal spinal position. Doctors found that Progressive Kyphosis of the cervical spine (a loss or reversing of the neck's curve) resulted in destruction of nerve fibers due to chronic compression of the spinal cord, similar to what happens with multiple sclerosis.[5]

Example of a Normal Cervical Curve or "Arc of Life"

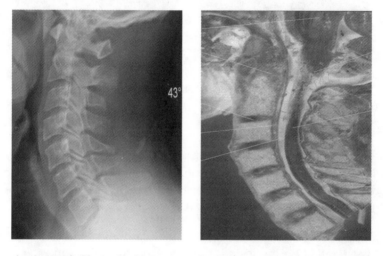

If you look at this X-ray, it shows a perfect curve, almost like the letter C. The dissection on the right shows the spinal cord inside. As you can see, because it's perfectly aligned, there is zero impingement on the spinal cord. So let me ask you a question: "How is this person functioning and healing?" That's right: 100 percent! As a result, how healthy are they? Right again: 100 percent.

Example of the Loss of the Arc of Life and the Degeneration That Follows

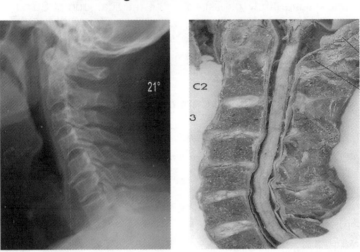

What do you see on the X-ray on the left? Absolutely no curve whatsoever, and if you look at the tiny three lower vertebrae and the spaces (discs) in between, you can see what happens as a result. This person has severe degenerative spine and disc disease.

If you look at the dissection on the right, you can see the spinal cord is degenerating on the inside. What do you think is happening to this person's health? What do you think is happening to this person's organs as a result of the power supply getting reduced or cut off?

A major problem here is that spinal misalignment, even this bad, may not be accompanied by pain at all. So the only way to really know if you have a problem like this is to get an X-ray.

Carol, 42 year-old female

Chiropractic evaluation:
Loss of cervical curve

Medical history:
Diabetes, Hypothyroid, Polycystic Ovarian Syndrome

Medications:
Metformin, Levothyroxin

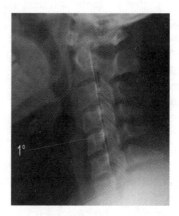

Real Arc of Life Story

Let's take a look at Carol, who is a 42 year-old female, diagnosed with Diabetes and polycystic ovarian syndrome for the last three years and suffers from a five-year history of hypothyroidism. When we initially met Carol, she was really in the dumps about her state of health. She was chronically tired, depressed, and hated her heavy menstrual cycles and pain associated with them.

I told her there was really only one solution and that was to get her body healing again. So we took an X-ray of her neck and found she had lost the curve. I told her, "It's like the water being cut off from the water supply that helps the plant to survive. The pinching on your spinal cord is causing your organs to barely survive, instead of thrive."

The plan to get started was immediate. Carol followed the Advanced Eating Plan and started to eliminate all sugars. As a result, she lost 12 pounds in her first week. We started to perform corrective chiropractic adjustments to restore the nerve supply, and she did her surge training exercises religiously. Within three months she had completely transformed her life and had reversed the diabetes and polycystic ovarian syndrome. How? Because the body doesn't need any help—just no interference!

Could That Hump in Your Back Be Killing You?

Look at what the in-depth medical literature says about chiropractic. A shocking 2004 study in the Journal of the American Geriatrics Society revealed that mortality could be predicted by the spine if it had subluxated to the point where there was an accentuation of the hump in the back, called Hyperkyphosis. An elite group of medical scientists found that as the curve in the middle back, or the Kyphosis, became greater than normal, death came sooner.[6] Are you hunched over? Go to the mirror right now or ask a family member or friend to look at your posture. Here's what to look for.

When you look at a person from the front, his spine should be straight. The head, shoulders, hips, and feet should be lined up. When you look at a person from the side, the ears should be back over the shoulders and the shoulders should be back over the pelvis.

The following are cases of abnormal posture.

- Head is visibly tilted, shifted, or rotated in one direction
- Head is jutted out in front of his chest and shoulders (forward-head syndrome)
- One hip is higher than the other, turned in one direction, or shifted to one side
- One shoulder is higher than the other, turned in one direction

In any case of abnormal posture, a person's central nervous system is experiencing interference or being damaged.

In addition to using the spinal X-rays and examination of the patient's posture to evaluate spine and nervous-system health, advances in technology have brought tests like EMG (Electromyography, which records the electrical activity of muscles), Thermography, Range of Motion, and muscle strength evaluations to give even more insight into the presence of neurological interference.

While not all Vertebral Subluxations cause major paralysis like Reeve suffered, any spinal interference at all detected by X-ray, posture, or any spinal test can wreak havoc on your health.

The big question chiropractors get is: "How did I possibly develop this type of problem if I didn't notice any pain or discomfort?"

Check any of the following causes of Vertebral Subluxation that apply to you:

- ❏ A challenging birth process (particularly with medical intervention)
- ❏ Falls and collisions as a child
- ❏ Sports injuries
- ❏ Auto accidents and other traumas
- ❏ Poor posture (computer work, long-distance driving, position at work, and the like)
- ❏ Improper sitting and sleeping positions (includes pillow and mattress problems)
- ❏ Any physical, mental, or chemical stress (chemical stress is caused primarily by processed foods, medications, and environmental toxins)
- ❏ Lack of exercise: weak or tight muscles

If you have answered yes to even one of these questions, then it's time to get a spinal evaluation right away. Because most people experience at least one of these causes, the presence of spinal misalignment (vertebral subluxation) is epidemic. The longer subluxation exists, the more degeneration and damage there is to the spine, central nervous system, and the organs they control.[7]

Aren't All Chiropractors the Same?

There are many kinds of chiropractors and most provide substantial value. In addition, their treatments are much safer than virtually any kind of medical treatment. However, as with all doctors, there are those who take their training to extremely high levels and who have differing levels of skills and areas of focus.

Chiropractic is a skill, so saying they're all the same is kind of like saying that all hairstylists are created equal. You've probably had some great haircuts and some really lousy haircuts. Training, coordination, technology, and a focus on spinal correction are all important factors when choosing someone to take care of your nervous system.

If your chiropractor has never taken a post X-ray to determine if the problem has been fixed by their care, then how did you know if it was actually corrected? More than likely, because you felt better. Sadly, every health problem, including a diseased spine, exists mostly without symptoms until later stages. Pain is the dangerous end of a problem, not the beginning or even the middle.

While some chiropractors choose to limit their scope of practice to treating pains or symptoms, others focus on overall health and longevity, starting with correcting and maintaining your spine to allow for Maximized Nerve Supply.

Testimonial — *Dan and Kristine Edwards*

You Mean My Spine is Degenerating?

Take the real-life case of Dan and Kristine Edwards, both of whom have seen chiropractors for years. However, when they came to one of our offices for an initial evaluation, both of their spines looked as if they had never been to a chiropractor. They had severe spinal decay and degeneration. So the common question arose, "What do you mean my spine is degenerating? I've been seeing chiropractors for years."

Even though they were visiting a chiropractor, they were only receiving adjustments when they had neck or back pain. Most of the time, if you feel pain, there's severe damage and inflammation that has already occurred. "But the chiropractic adjustments made us feel better," Kristine proclaimed.

The reality is, however, that because Dan and Kristine had never had the problems in their spines corrected and then strengthened and maintained those corrections, their spines were in worse shape than ever. It was as if they'd never had a single adjustment. Additionally, it was why their health problems continued to come back.

The seemingly miraculous stories that you have read about in this book and the thousands more you can discover in our offices or view on our Web sites were initiated by chiropractors focusing on correction.

Testimonial — *Mary Shnedler, 58 years old*

I Even Went to Say Good-bye to My Kids

The trouble started in June of 1993. That's when my car rolled four times down a hill. During that long, terrifying tumble, I hit my head pretty hard and broke my tailbone. When I woke up, I couldn't remember who I was, where I lived, or what my phone number was. My lefts were rights, my Ps were Bs and my sixes were nines. I went to 14 different specialists. They gave me so many pain pills that my liver started to deteriorate. Soon I was taking Prozac for depression. After a year, my body was still so wracked with pain that they sent me to an internist. Many tests later, he said I had fibromyalgia. I have lived with this pain on and off ever since.

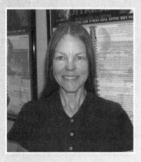

Then another catastrophe hit. In October 2007, I fell down the stairs in my house. The MRI showed a crushed vertebra. Doctors put me on more pain medicine, some of which upset my system. I got shots for pain and inflammation. Before long, I had lost some feeling in my right shoulder and my right fingers started to turn purple. I couldn't comb my hair, brush my teeth, or lift my arm high enough to clean under my arms. I thought I was dying. My whole body seemed to lock up on me with my muscles in knots. I lost weight and muscle. I was so tired and weak that I couldn't work. I would lie in bed barely moving. When I did move, pain shot through my body as if cut by a knife. If my husband moved the sheets, I recoiled in pain. Not even morphine could ease my pain. I couldn't sleep or think straight. My husband had to help me dress. I needed a cane or walker to get around. I couldn't bend over to pick things up off the floor. I cried a lot. I seriously wondered if I was going crazy.

With all those drugs in my system, I developed a heart murmur. My pulse rate fluctuated and my heart raced. Naturally, the cardiologist put me on medicine for that as well. I had to take thyroid medication too. Before I found Maximized Living, I truly thought my life was coming to an end. I had lost all hope. I even went to say good-bye to my kids. Thank God I found another way.

The sad thing was that I had been married to a chiropractor for 16 years and had gone to several chiropractors ever since my first accident. But none of them knew how to resolve my problems—until I learned about Maximized Living. No other medical doctor or chiropractor I have known was able to heal me the way Maximized Living doctors did.

My life began again in October 2008, when I attended a Maximized Living Seminar at our church. I was impressed by the focus on overall health. They talked about how corrective chiropractic could actually cure long-term spinal misalignments. He said that your body can heal itself if you unblock the nervous system, eat well, and exercise. I knew right away I desperately needed his help.

With the help of Maximized Living, my pain began to go away and I slowly stopped taking my pain medications. Now I am drug-free. I don't even need the thyroid pills I took for years. My heart is also fine without medication.

Clinical Results with Chronic Fatigue and Fibromyalgia in a Patient Who Had Seen Doctors and Chiropractors for Years

Neil had seen a chiropractor for over five years and an endless array of other medical specialists. Yet, he still suffered with severe migraine headaches, debilitating neck pain, and was recently diagnosed with fibromyalgia and chronic fatigue syndrome.

Neil walked into one of our offices and proclaimed, "I am just sick and tired of being sick and tired, and I don't want to be on this medication anymore. It's making me worse!"

He had a grocery bag full of medications that he was taking. He needed help desperately. Like many patients, he remarked, "But you don't understand, I've been to chiropractors before and it didn't help. How are you different?" Our extensive evaluation revealed that he had no arc in his neck. I told him, "No matter what you do, nothing will make a difference in your health unless your body is healing first, and the only way you will get healing is if we get your brain connected to your body. Your body doesn't need any help—just no interference. We need to get your arc back."

Desperate for help, Neil focused on his care. He never missed his appointments and did all of the simple exercises. In a short amount of time, post X-rays of his neck showed the curve in his neck was restored. With 100 percent function and 100 percent healing, he was pain free and able to stop taking all medications.

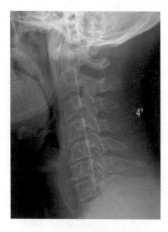 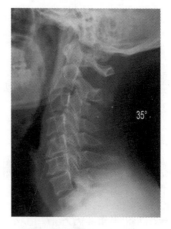

NEIL BEFORE CARE   **NEIL'S POST X-RAY**
No Arc of Life & spinal decay   *Near normal Arc of Life*
(Previously had five years of chiropractic)

Safety of Spinal Correction Is Unparalleled in Health Care

Unlike many medical procedures, chiropractic adjustments are incredibly safe. In a study reported in Spine Journal in October 2007 of more than 19,700 patients who underwent more than 50,000 cervical spine adjustments, a team of researchers concluded that the risk of having a serious adverse event from "getting your neck cracked" is none. The manipulation technique at the focus of this safety study was defined as the application of high-velocity/low-amplitude or mechanically assisted thrust to the cervical spine. Patients were followed and any adverse symptoms were recorded immediately, up to seven days after treatment. There were no reports of serious adverse events.[8]

This and many other studies show why chiropractors pay a fraction of a fraction for malpractice, compared to medical doctors. It's so safe that, while MDs pay $20,000 to $100,00 for malpractice insurance, chiropractors have malpractice insurance that's far cheaper than your car insurance. Why? Because insurance companies go by computer-generated facts about safety, not myths.

Completing Step 3: What Should I Do Now?

Now that we've shown you that the single most important healing mechanism in your body is your nervous system, the time to act is now.

"Remember, a real decision is measured by the fact you've taken new action. If there's no action, you haven't truly decided."[9]

—— *Anthony Robbins*

To be headed to the cruise ship and avoid wheelchairs, walkers, and dependence on others, it's urgent that you get yourself and your family in for spinal evaluations by a corrective-care chiropractor—even if you've had an evaluation by a chiropractor before. You can go to **www.maximizedliving.com** to the "Find a Doctor" section to find the nearest doctor in your area.

Max-Mind Moment

Remember Who You Are

This Maximized Moment may contain the number-one thing you must do to reach your potential and live the abundant life you were created to live. Perhaps the best way to sum up the Maximized Mind is by saying, "Remember who you are!"

Who are you? You are the most mind-boggling, creative, healing machine that has ever been created. The power inside of you knew how to take two cells in your mother's womb and turn them into an eating, breathing, pooping, seventy-trillion-celled baby in nine months! That power has never left you. You're still powerful. That power has remained on the job, replacing fifty thousand cells per second, every second that you draw a breath. With this incredible power inside of you, there is a big responsibility to take care of it and not forget about it.

The key to remembering who you are is listening to the right people. Every day, people are telling you (and your kids) who they think you are—something small, weak, and being overpowered by your environment and your circumstances.

Who are you listening to? Are you listening to the swine flu fear mongers on the news telling you that you are going to die? Are you listening to the drug company ads telling you that you are somehow broken or too weak to heal yourself? Are you listening to the doctors who, for decades, told you mammograms and hormone replacement therapy were a good idea until they just realized that they can actually cause cancer?

A patient of ours babysits the daughter of a medical doctor who works for Kaiser Permanente. When the patient went to take care of the doctor's eighteen-month-old daughter, guess what the baby girl was drinking in her sippy cup? Diet Coke! The "expert on health" was giving her own one year-old Diet Coke—an artificially colored, artificially flavored black liquid! This is so antihealth it's not worth even describing. Yet, this isn't meant to speak badly about the doctor. The doctor just didn't know any better. That is, until our patient decided to educate her.

The point is that you have to be very careful about who you listen to. If you've had some health struggles or fallen off course, join the club! Don't give in when you hit some adversity. There are two important quotes to remember:

1. "Fatigue makes cowards of us all." You only get fatigued if you listen to the people filling you with death and fear. You were not created to function in fear.

2. "There is a way that seems right to a man but in the end leads to death" (Proverbs 14:12). It may be common, but it may also be abnormal. When a billion people believe in a bad idea, it's still a bad idea! Please don't perish because you lack the knowledge of who you really are. Be careful who you listen to. Remember who you are!

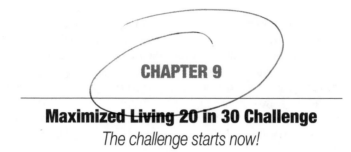

CHAPTER 9

Maximized Living 20 in 30 Challenge
The challenge starts now!

Take a look at the calendar. How would you like to be 20 pounds lighter one month from now? Does that sound too good to be true? We have seen thousands of people lose 20 pounds in 30 days with the plan you have in front of you. You've met many of them in this book. It is so powerful because it combines the true science of weight loss (hormones) and a plan that people can actually DO! We aren't asking you to eat Melba toast and celery sticks or starve yourself. We aren't asking you to join an expensive gym or spend hours on the treadmill. No more counting calories or footsteps! The meals on the plan are filling and delicious and the fat burning exercise can be done in the time it takes to make a cup of coffee. The best part is that you will regulate your hormones so that you build muscle and burn fat around the clock, not just while you're exercising.

You'll get daily tips to win the biggest battle of all- the one that goes on between your ears. Science shows that it only takes 21 days to form a new habit, so the healthy habits you form in the next month will be with you for the rest of your life.

This will be the biggest factor in your success- prepare to win! When your old habits try to creep back in, it is vital to have the right foods in your house so that you don't cave in because you weren't prepared. This is your shopping day. At the back of the book, you'll find your shopping lists for each week. We recommend that you do this on a Sunday and start your challenge on Monday. You'll have the right foods to fuel your body, stay full and stay on track.

One secret to success is the smoothies that you will be drinking. They are a fast, tasty way to make sure you are getting what you need and staying on track. The recipe calls for whey protein and our families use the **Perfect Protein**® from Maximized Living. Most protein powders on the market today have low quality, hydrolyzed proteins and are filled with dangerous artificial sweeteners like aspartame and sucralose. We also don't recommend soy protein for a variety of reasons. Soy protein isolate has been shown to interfere with immune and hormone function.

Whey protein is nature's richest source of biologically available protein, complete with all 22 essential amino acids. Whey protein contains powerful immune boosters and helps to synthesize antioxidants necessary for detoxification. Studies by Dr. Donald Layman, a professor at the University of Illinois, have highlighted the role of the amino acid Leucine in sculpting your body. High quality whey protein is rich in Leucine to help preserve lean muscle tissue while promoting fat loss. Whey protein contains more Leucine than rice protein, egg protein and soy protein.

According to the Mayo clinic, whey protein helps stabilize blood sugar levels by slowing the absorption of glucose into the bloodstream. This in turn reduces hunger by lowering insulin levels and making it easier for your body to burn fat. You simply cannot beat whey protein.

Most of the whey protein you see in stores has been high temperature processed, which basically kills the health producing qualities of when. **Perfect Protein**® comes from naturally raised, grass-fed cows that have never been injected with antibiotics or hormones. Vital enzymes and nutrients remain intact through low temperature delicate filtration.

MAXIMIZED LIVING 20 in 30 MEAL PLAN – *(Week 1 & 3)*

Monday	Tuesday	Wednesday	Thursday	Friday	Saturday	Sunday
Breakfast: Cheesy Scrambled eggs with cheddar cheese Use almond milk to mix eggs	**Breakfast:** 1 cup Greek yogurt with fresh berries and coconut-Xylitol or Stevia to taste	**Breakfast:** Perfect French Vanilla Smoothie	**Breakfast:** Berry Blast Smoothie	**Breakfast:** Chocolate Power Smoothie	**Breakfast:** Perfect French Vanilla smoothie	**Breakfast:** Scrambled Eggs with 2 sliced turkey bacon
Snack: 1/2 cup raw almonds	**Snack:** 3 to 5 celery sticks with 1/2 cup hummus	**Snack:** 3 to 5 sticks celery filled with almond butter	**Snack:** 1/2 cup pumpkin seeds	**Snack:** Vegetable sticks of your choice with 1/2 cup hummus	**Snack:** 1/2 cup raw nuts and seeds	**Snack:** 1 cup Greek yogurt with 2 tbs chopped pistachios and 2 tbs cacao nibs-Xylitol or Stevia to taste Let cacao nibs sit In yogurt for 15 minutes to soften up and then add pistachios
Lunch: Green Salad with grilled or baked chicken breast with 1/4 cup olive oil and 3 tablespoons white or balsamic vinegar	**Lunch:** Left over Easy Advanced Plan Chili	**Lunch:** Green salad with baked or grilled salmon and 1/4 cup olive oil and 3 tbs balsamic or while vinegar	**Lunch:** Left over black bean soup	**Lunch:** Left over Vegetable Beef Soup	**Lunch:** Chicken Salad	**Lunch:** Grilled Chicken Breast, black beans and salsa
Snack: 3 to 5 celery sticks with 1/2 cup hummus	**Snack:** 1/2 cup raw walnuts	**Snack:** 8 to 10 Celery, carrot and pepper sticks with 1/2 guacamole	**Snack:** 1/2 cup Greek yogurt with fresh berries and sliced almonds-Xylitol or Stevia to taste	**Snack:** Granny Smith apple with 1/4 cup almond butter	**Snack:** 1 or 2 Boiled Eggs	**Snack:** Granny Smith Apple with 1/4 cup almond butter
Dinner: Easy Advanced Plan Chili	**Dinner:** Grass fed steak Broccoli and cauliflower Steamed or roasted. Can add brussel sprouts or other vegetables	**Dinner:** Black Bean Fiesta Soup	**Dinner:** Mom's Vegetable Beef Soup	**Dinner:** Jamie's Chicken stir Fry	**Dinner:** Southwest Cod or Halibut Mashed faux-potatoes Green Salad	**Dinner:** TastyTeriyaki Salmon Broccoli

MAXIMIZED LIVING 20 in 30 MEAL PLAN – *(Week 2 & 4)*

Monday	Tuesday	Wednesday	Thursday	Friday	Saturday	Sunday
Breakfast: Perfect French Vanilla Smoothie Add greens (optional) **Snack:** 1/2 cup raw almonds **Lunch:** Green salad with grilled or baked chicken breast with 1/4 cup olive oil and 3 tbs balsamic vinegar **Snack:** 3 to 5 celery sticks with 1/2 cup hummus **Dinner:** Classic Pot Roast with Sauerkraut and optional green salad	**Breakfast:** Chocolate Power Smoothie Add greens (optional) **Snack:** 1 or 2 Boiled Eggs **Lunch:** Leftover pot roast **Snack:** 1/2 cup raw almonds **Dinner:** Juicy Grilled Steak with Bernaise sauce Sauteed pinach, Kale, or Broccoli Save some beef if you want for Sunday's lunch	**Breakfast:** Berry Blast Smoothie Add greens (optional) **Snack:** 3 to 5 celery sticks filled with almond butter **Lunch:** Chicken salad (Make 1/4 the recipe for 1) **Snack:** 1/2 cup walnuts **Dinner:** Black Bean Fiesta Soup	**Breakfast:** Perfect French Vanilla Smoothie Add greens (optional) **Snack:** 1/2 cup pumpkin seeds **Lunch:** Leftover Black Bean Fiesta Soup **Snack:** 1 or 2 Boiled Eggs **Dinner:** Jamie's Chicken Stir Fry	**Breakfast:** Unsweetend Greek yogurt and blueberries with 2 tbs Sliced almonds- Xylitol or Stevia to taste **Snack:** Carrot, celery and bell pepper strips w/ 1/2 cup hummus **Lunch:** Green Salad w/ baked or grilled salmon with 1/4 cup olive oil and 3 tbs balsamic vinegar **Snack:** 5 Celery sticks with 1/2 cup hummus **Dinner:** Vivian's Shepherd's Pie	**Breakfast:** Chocolate Power Smoothie Add greens (optional) **Snack:** 1/2 cup walnuts **Lunch:** Leftover Shepherd's Pie **Snack:** 1 or 2 Boiled Eggs **Dinner:** Baked Cod or Halibut Mashed faux-pota- toes Green Salad	**Breakfast:** Berry Blast Smoothie Add greens (optional) **Snack:** 5 Celery or broccoli sticks with 1/2 cup hummus **Lunch:** Chinese cabbage salad with chicken or sliced beef **Snack:** 1/2 cup raw almonds **Dinner:** Chicken Coconut Curry

Shopping Success Tips:

- Most ingredients used in the recipes can be found at your local grocery store in the organic or natural section.
- While organic fruits and vegetables are best, they are not necessary if you have budget constraints.
- For some items like quality grass-fed or free-range meat or raw cheeses, you may have to locate your nearest health food store.

USE THIS	NOT THIS
Coconut Oil, Olive Oil	Pam, Crisco, Vegetable Oil, Canola Oil
Homemade Dressings Made With Vinegar, Oil, and Seasonings	Store Bought Salad Dressings (high in sugar)
Bragg's Liquid Aminos	Soy Sauce
Stevia/Xylitol	Sugar
Vegenaise (grapeseed)	Mayo/Miracle Whip
Flax/Almond/ Coconut Flour	Regular Flour
Zevia Pop Natural Organic Soda	Regular Sodas

Making the Meal Plan Work for You:

- Feel free to interchange the meals if you don't want something on a particular day. Always use breakfast as breakfast but the lunches and dinners are interchangeable. Most of the recipes freeze very well and make great lunches or dinners for later. If you don't like a particular dish you don't have to make it again. Use something else on the plan in its place. This is not a diet! It's the basis of an eating plan that will keep you healthy and trim to your 120th birthday!

- A good snack is canned chickpeas. Rinse well and salt to taste with good salt and eat like peanuts. Don't overdo it-just twice a week.

- You can also add a handful of spinach or kale to any smoothie. You can't taste it but you get all that good raw nutrition.

- Make a pitcher of lemonade to keep in your refrigerator. Just squeeze lemons, add water and xylitol or Stevia to taste. This will help curb any "sweet tooth" cravings.

"Out To Dinner" Tips & Ordering Ideas:

- Order Water, almost all other options likely contain sugar.

- Always order, "Sauce on the side." Again, many/all will contain sugar.

- Take Stevia or Xylitol packets with you if you order tea or coffee.

  - Don't feel like you have to finish everything. Restaurants give you extremely large portions. Most meals are 2-3 times bigger than a normal serving size. Save 1/2 for lunch the next day or split the meal with someone else.

  - Skip the bread and butter before your meal. In fact, ask them to not even bring it to the table.

- **Breakfast:**
- Vegetable Omelets with a cup of berries (hold hashbrowns/ breads)

- **Lunch:**
- Salads! (replace the salad dressing with salsa or oil/vinegar)
- Burrito place: do a burrito bowl, hold the tortilla.

- **Italian:**
- Order grilled chicken pasta and hold pasta, double the veggies.
- Order the entrée with chicken, beef, etc, hold the starch and double the veggies.
- Salad with Olive Oil and Balsamic Vinegar. Almost all restaurants have Olive Oil and vinegar if you ask for it.

- **Mexican:**
- Order fajitas without tortillas. You still get all the flavor without the grains.
- Ask if the restaurant has sliced jicama to dip in salsa/guacamole (as an alternative to chips).

- **Asian:**
- Order steamed vegetables in place of fried/stir fry vegetables
- Hold the rice, try a seaweed salad!
- Sushi is a great option, just hold the rice or do lettuce wraps.

- **Bar/Grill:**
- Order a burger with lettuce wrap bun or no bun. Veggies instead of fries.
- Add black beans and avocados for a more filling side salad.
- Order 2 sides of vegetables, instead of 1 starch and 1 vegetable.

Day 1
Your Assessment: *The Man or Woman in Your Mirror*

"Wherever you go, there you are."

—*Author Unknown*

So, here is your action step: don't read another sentence until you find a mirror and answer these questions.

Man or woman in the mirror: What's your number? The first step to changing is finding out where you are. Take the following test to find out how close you are to the cruise ship or nursing home. You will re-take the test after 28 days to see your progress.

Adult Body Mass Index

$$BMI = \left[\frac{Weight\ (pounds)}{Height\ (inches)^2} \right] \times 703$$

	WEIGHT IN POUNDS													
	120	130	140	150	160	170	180	190	200	210	220	230	240	250
4'-6"	29	31	34	36	39	41	43	46	48	51	53	56	58	60
4'-8"	27	29	31	34	36	38	40	43	45	47	49	52	54	56
4'-10"	25	27	29	31	34	36	38	40	42	44	46	48	50	52
5'-0"	23	25	27	29	31	33	35	37	39	41	43	45	47	49
5'-2"	22	24	26	27	29	31	33	35	37	38	40	42	44	46
5'-4"	21	22	24	26	28	29	31	33	34	36	38	40	41	43
5'-6"	19	21	23	24	26	27	29	31	32	34	36	37	39	40
5'-8"	18	20	21	23	24	26	27	29	30	32	34	35	37	38
5'-10"	17	19	20	22	23	24	26	27	29	30	32	33	35	36
6'-0"	16	18	19	20	22	23	24	26	27	28	30	31	33	34
6'-2"	15	17	18	19	21	22	23	24	26	27	28	30	31	32
6'-4"	15	16	17	18	20	21	22	23	24	26	27	28	29	30
6'-6"	14	15	16	17	19	20	21	22	23	24	25	27	28	29
6'-8"	13	14	15	17	18	19	20	21	22	23	24	25	26	28

HEIGHT IN FEET & INCHES

■ Healthy Weight   ■ Overweight   ■ Obese

	10 points	5 points	0 points
What's your BMI?	Less than 24	25-29	Over 30
What's your waist to hip ratio? (Waist is measured 1 in above navel, hips at widest point of buttocks)	.95 or below for men .80 or below for women	.96 to 1.0 for men .81 to .85 for women	1.0+ for men .85+ for women
How many medications are you taking?	0	1-2	More than 2
How many days a week do you skip breakfast?	0	1-2	More than 2
How many meals per week do you eat fast food?	0	1-2	More than 2
What is your resting pulse? (Beats per minute)	Less than 70	71-83	Over 83
How many times per week do you exercise?	More than 3	1-2	None
How many flu shots have you gotten?	Never	1-2	More than 2
How many sodas or sweetened beverages (tea, sports drinks, etc) do you drink per week?	0	1-2	More than 2
How many hours per night do you sleep?	8 or more	7	Less than 7

Where are you headed?
0-20 Sprinting towards the nursing home
21-40 It's time to get moving now
41-60 Assess your weak areas and get a plan
61-80 Stay consistent and keep improving
81-100 Keep it up and we'll see you on the cruise ship

Mandatory 1st step: Get an accountability partner. Twice the help equals twice the results. It can be your spouse, co-worker or friend. Write down your goals you want to achieve for the challenge and exchange them with your partner.

Eating Plan:

Breakfast:
Cheesy Eggs

Snack:
1/2 cup raw almonds

Lunch:
Chicken Breast Salad with 1/4 cup Olive Oil and 3 tablespoons White or Balsamic Vinegar

Snack:
3 to 5 celery sticks with 1/2 cup hummus

Dinner:
Easy Advanced Plan Chili

If you have the Max T3 DVD's, your daily workout will be listed in each day of the challenge. We have seen the best results if you have the DVD's, so that you can follow along with the workouts in the comfort of your own home. If you don't have the DVD's, you can pick your surge exercises from Chapter 7 and do a surge cycle each day or your choice.

Max T3: Superfast Workout 1 – Upper Body

Day 2
Your Big Why

It's time for you to get a bigger Why. Right now, we want you to come up with the most compelling reason that you can for taking control of your health. If you want to lose weight just to look good in your bathing suit, that is not a big enough Why. If you want to lose weight because you want to be around to pass your wisdom on to your grandchildren at their weddings, now you are getting somewhere. Write down your Big Why so that you can refer to it every day for the next thirty days.

My Big Why:

_____

_____

Take time now to think about your Big Why. What's most important to you? How do you see your future? How could an improved life, mind, body, and soul help you achieve your dreams?

Eating Plan:

Breakfast:
1 cup Greek yogurt with fresh berries and coconut-Xylitol or Stevia to taste

Snack:
3 to 5 celery sticks with 1/2 cup hummus

Lunch:
Left over Easy Advanced Plan Chili

Snack:
1/2 cup raw walnuts

Dinner:
Grass fed steak
Broccoli and cauliflower

Toxicity Tip: Read food (and gum) labels and eliminate all artificial sweeteners, including Aspartame and Sucralose and switch to Stevia or Xylitol.

Max T3: Superfast Workout 2 – Lower Body

Day 3
Max Mind:

Changing Your Beliefs: The Fast Track to Success

The biggest reason why you may have failed in the past is because you don't believe you can actually reach your goals and live the life you've always dreamed about. You try something new, then an old limiting belief shows up and decides, "I'll never be able to really have that anyway, so I might as well go back to how I was living before." The reality is, change scares us and scares others around us.

So how do you get over your limiting belief and move in the directions of your dreams? First you have to identify the limiting belief and create a new belief. The following is an exercise to help you do that.

1. Write down a belief that is holding you back.
Some examples of limiting beliefs are: "I'm too old to lose weight," "I have bad genes, so I have to be on this medication forever," "I don't have enough time to workout," "I'm too lazy," or "I never win at anything."

_____

_____

_____

_____

2. Now cross out that old belief and write a new empowering belief.
For example, cross out "I'm too old to lose weight" and change it to "I can lose weight easily and quickly." Cross out "I don't have enough time to work out" and change it to "I make time to work out every day because I'm worth it." Cross out "I hate health food" and change it to "I'm constantly finding easy ways to prepare delicious foods that taste better than junk food and make me feel good instead of sick when I eat them."

In order to retrain your brain, you need to say this new affirmation three times in the morning and three times before bed for thirty days. It takes that long to program a new belief. So once you've identified your limiting belief, as soon as that old belief comes up, stop in the middle of thinking it and say the new empowering belief. For example, "I'm too old... No, I am not too old. I can lose weight easily and quickly!"

The stronger and more dominant the new picture of yourself is in your mind, the faster the new belief forms and the more powerful the process is.

_____

_____

_____

_____

Once this new belief becomes a part of you, your mind will start "correcting for the mistake," but in a way that moves you closer to your goals. If you truly believe that you are a person that makes good food choices, you will look at that candy bar and say, "That's not me." This is where things get fun!

You may consider yourself a hopeless case. We have patients who think they are genetically doomed to have certain diseases or that their health has deteriorated too far to recover, but the facts prove them completely wrong. The International Agency for Research on Cancer and the World Health Organization have concluded that 80 percent of all cancers are attributed to lifestyle, not genetics.[2] And this is a conservative number. Other studies reveal that as little as two percent of all diseases and conditions have anything to do with genetics or so-called "bad luck."[3] In other words, as much as 98 percent of all body types, conditions, and disease are due all or in part to lifestyle.

Studies have shown that many people who live 100 years have genes that are supposedly high risk for disease and early death.[4] This shows that almost everybody can do something to stay healthy—no matter who their grandparents are.

You are hearing a lot of "you can't" messages from your doctor, the news, and maybe your aunt Sally, but we're here to tell you that you can! You are not a victim of bad genes or bad luck. You have more potential inside of you than you can imagine. The biggest shame that we see as doctors is when people settle for less than their potential. They rationalize being sick and feeling bad. But you hold the key to your health future, and our specialty is showing you how to use that key.

Do you ever say any of these things?
- Everyone has headaches!
- My insomnia isn't as bad as my wife's!
- I'm not really that tired!
- Sure, I've slowed down and put on some weight. I'm over thirty, and that's what happens.

You know what? Everyone doesn't have headaches. Any insomnia stinks no matter how bad someone else has it. Tired is just tired. There are people up to eighty and ninety years old with abs and who run marathons! You were never meant to fall apart, degenerate, and feel old and tired. You have the most incredible healing, regenerating power on Planet Earth inside of you! Stop settling for anything less than the energy, vitality, and abundant health that you were designed for!

Whatever you've been told about yourself or your abilities is not the truth. It may be the truth you believe, but you don't have to hold on to it.

Eating Plan:

Breakfast:
Perfect French Vanilla Smoothie

Snack:
3 to 5 sticks celery filled with Almond Butter

Lunch:
Salmon Salad with 1/4 cup Olive Oil and 3 Tbs. Balsamic or White Vinegar

Snack:
8 to 10 assorted veggie sticks with 1/2 guacamole

Dinner:
Black Bean Fiesta Soup

Max T3: Superfast Workout 3 - Core

Day 4

Max Mind: Creating an incentive is a powerful way to achieve your goals. Share your commitments with your accountability partner and if you don't fulfill your commitment, give them permission to email your friends your failed results. Pressure's on!

Eating Plan:

Breakfast:
Berry Blast Smoothie

Snack:
1/2 cup Pumpkin Seeds

Lunch:
Left over Black Bean Fiesta Soup

Snack:
1/2 cup Greek yogurt with fresh berries and sliced almonds-Xylitol or Stevia to taste

Dinner:
Old Fashioned Vegetable Beef Soup

Toxicity Tip: Switch to Extra Virgin Olive Oil and/or Coconut Oil. Throw out foods containing hydrogenated or partially hydrogenated oils, including Corn Oil, Canola Oil, Vegetable Oil, Soybean Oil and Safflower Oil, (salad dressings etc.).

Max T3: Superfast Workout 4 – Surge

Day 5

Max Mind: Some people are motivated by pleasure or pain. Decide which one you are! Create an action step for reaching your goal, either give yourself something amazing for your efforts ie a vacation or spa day. Or force yourself to do something that scares you, ie. Run a marathon.

Eating Plan:

Breakfast:
Chocolate Power Smoothie

Snack:
Veggie Sticks with ranch dressing

Lunch:
Left over Old Fashioned Vegetable Beef Soup

Snack:
Granny Smith apple with 1/2 cup Almond Butter

Dinner:
Jamie's Chicken Stir Fry

Max T3: Superfast Workout 5 – Upper Body

Day 6

Max Mind: Don't forget to journal everything you eat from here forward. Writing it down makes you 3 times more accountable to what goes in your mouth.

Eating Plan:

Breakfast:
Perfect French Vanilla Smoothie

Snack:
1/2 cup raw nuts and seeds

Lunch:
Chicken Breast Salad with 1/4 cup Olive Oil and 3 Tbs. Balsamic Vinegar

Snack:
Boiled Egg

Dinner:
South West Cod or Halibut
Mashed faux-potatoes
Green Salad

Toxicity Tip: Clean water equals clean body! Switch your bottled water to distilled or reverse osmosis. You can also buy a water filter for your house. We recommend reverse osmosis or a good carbon block filter.

Max T3: Superfast Workout 6 – Lower Body

Day 7

Max Mind: Preparation! Preparation! Preparation! If you fail to plan, you are planning to fail! Prepare your meals for the week on Saturday or Sunday and know exactly when you are exercising!

Eating Plan:

Breakfast:
Scrambled Eggs with 2 slices turkey bacon

Snack:
1 cup Greek yogurt with 2 Tbs. chopped pistachios and 2 Tbs. Cacao nibs-Xylitol or Stevia to taste

Lunch:
Grilled Chicken Breast with black beans and salsa

Snack:
Granny Smith Apple with 1/2 cup Almond Butter

Dinner:
Tasty Teriyaki Salmon
Broccoli

Max T3: REST!

Day 8

Max Mind: Review your Big Why. Really get a vision of how it looks when you get there. How does it make you feel? When it gets tough this week (and it will) get that feeling back and remember WHY you are doing this!

Eating Plan:

Breakfast:
Perfect French Vanilla Smoothie

Snack:
1/2 cup raw almonds

Lunch:
Chicken Breast Salad with 1/4 cup Olive Oil and 3 Tbs. Balsamic Vinegar

Snack:
3 to 5 celery sticks with 1/2 cup hummus

Dinner:
Classic Pot Roast with Sauerkraut

Max T3: Fast Workout 7 – Upper Body

Day 9

Max Mind: Stop thinking "It's too hard". Being in a body that does not make you feel your absolute best is hard. You can do this.

Eating Plan:

Breakfast:
Chocolate Power Smoothie

Snack:
Boiled Egg

Lunch:
Leftover Classic Pot Roast

Snack:
1/2 cup raw almonds

Dinner:
Juicy Grilled Steak with Bernaise sauce sautéed Spinach, Kale, or Broccoli

Toxicity Tip: Boost your Glutathione levels. Glutathione is your body's best defense against the toxins and bombard you each day. You can boost your Glutathione levels by eating cruciferous vegetables like broccoli and Brussels sprouts. Un-denatured whey protein like the **Perfect Protein®** from Maximized Living in your smoothie is an even better way to dramatically decrease your risk of toxin related diseases!

Max T3: Fast Workout 8 – Lower Body

Day 10

Max Mind: If you feel that you have no time to exercise, REMEMBER it's only 12 minutes! In the time it takes to park your car at Starbucks, stand in line, order your latte and get back in your car, you could be DONE with your exercise for the week that turned your body into a fat burning machine.

Eating Plan:

Breakfast:
Berry Blast Smoothie

Snack:
3 to 5 celery sticks filled with Almond Butter

Lunch:
Chicken Breast Salad with 1/4 cup Olive Oil and 3 Tbs. Balsamic Vinegar

Snack:
1/2 cup walnuts

Dinner:
Black Bean Fiesta Soup

Max T3: Fast Workout 9 – Core

Day 11

Max Mind: Don't think "I messed up so I'll just eat whatever I want now". You are not on a diet and you are making healthy choices every day and you should be proud of the changes you made this far. If you haven't done everything perfect, you are still better off than 99% of the people you know! The fact that you are reading this means that you are doing better than you think you are.

Eating Plan:

Breakfast:
Perfect French Vanilla Smoothie

Snack:
1/2 cup Pumpkin Seeds

Lunch:
Leftover Healthy Black Bean Soup

Snack:
Boiled Egg

Dinner:
Jamie's Chicken Stir Fry

Toxicity Tip: Eliminate all Teflon cookware....danger! Switch to stainless steel, cast iron or micro-ceramic cookware.

Max T3: Fast Workout 10 – Surge

Day 12

Max Mind: Warning: Don't go shopping when you are hungry, somehow your favorite snack ends up in the cart. You'll be surprised at the healthier choices you make when you shop when you are satisfied.

Eating Plan:

Breakfast:
Unsweetened Greek yogurt and blueberries with 2 Tbs. Sliced almonds – Xylitol or Stevia to taste

Snack:
Veggie sticks with 1/2 cup hummus

Lunch:
Salmon Salad with 1/4 cup Olive Oil and 3 Tbs. Balsamic Vinegar

Snack:
Celery sticks with hummus

Dinner:
Vivian's Shepherd's Pie

Max T3: Fast Workout 11 – Upper Body

Day 13

Max Mind: You've probably said "I should get involved in other activities and refrain from eating this but I just don't care". It's true that you don't care at that moment, but pretty soon you're going to feel really bad that you ate that, and when you get on the scale you will care very much.

Eating Plan:

Breakfast:
Chocolate Power Smoothie

Snack:
1/2 cup walnuts

Lunch:
Leftover Pellow's Shepherd's Pie

Snack:
Boiled Egg

Dinner:
Quick Baked Cod or Halibut
Mashed faux-potatoes
Green Salad

Toxicity Tip: The best all natural cleaner is equal part water and vinegar in spray bottle for an intense cleaning solution for countertops, sinks and bathtubs.

Max T3: Fast Workout 12 – Lower Body

Day 14

Max Mind: Failing to plan is planning to fail. Get your shopping done today!

Eating Plan:

Breakfast:
Berry Blast Smoothie

Snack:
Celery sticks with 1/2 cup hummus

Lunch:
Chinese cabbage salad with chicken

Snack:
1/2 cup raw almonds

Dinner:
Chicken Coconut Curry

Max T3: REST!

Day 15

Mind: Spend five minutes picturing your Big Why. Is it getting more real to you now? You are well on your way to achieving your vision-keep up the good work.

Eating Plan:

Breakfast:
Cheesy Eggs

Snack:
1/2 cup raw almonds

Lunch:
Chicken Breast Salad with 1/4 cup Olive Oil and 3 tablespoons White or Balsamic Vinegar

Snack:
3 to 5 celery sticks with 1/2 cup hummus

Dinner:
Easy Advanced Plan Chili

Max T3: Superfast Workout 1 – Upper Body

Day 16

Max Mind: Stay on track! At this point you may think that you don't need to schedule meals, but eating how you have been eating has not worked out, so you sticking to scheduled eating gives you the freedom from emotional eating!

Eating Plan:

Breakfast:
1 cup Greek yogurt with fresh berries and coconut-Xylitol or Stevia to taste

Snack:
3 to 5 celery sticks with 1/2 cup hummus

Lunch:
Left over Easy Advanced Plan Chili

Snack:
1/2 cup raw walnuts

Dinner:
Grass fed steak
Broccoli and cauliflower

Toxicity Tip: For amazing toxic free face wash, that even removes makeup, mix Almond Oil and a 1/2 tsp. of honey.

Max T3: Superfast Workout 2 – Lower Body

Day 17

Max Mind: You are starting to see results so stay positive. Don't tell yourself "I'm not going to be happy until your goals are reached". You can choose to be happy now, dwelling on unhappiness is what got you into this mess. Be happy with you results now and continue to make good choices.

Eating Plan:

Breakfast:
Perfect French Vanilla Smoothie

Snack:
3 to 5 sticks celery filled with Almond Butter

Lunch:
Salmon Salad and 1/4 cup Olive Oil and 3 Tbs. Balsamic or While Vinegar

Snack:
8 to 10 assorted veggie sticks with 1/2 cup guacamole

Dinner:
Black Bean Fiesta Soup

Max T3: Superfast Workout 3 – Core

Day 18

Max Mind: If you've been sticking to the plan so far, your friends and family are probably looking at you like you are a little crazy with all this "health stuff." That's a good thing. The way the world is going right now, you don't want to be normal. Mark Twain said, "When you find yourself on the side of the majority, it's time to pause and reflect." Weird is good!

Eating Plan:

Breakfast:
Berry Blast Smoothie

Snack:
1/2 cup Pumpkin Seeds

Lunch:
Left over Healthy Black Bean Soup

Snack:
1/2 cup Greek yogurt with fresh berries and sliced almonds-Xylitol or Stevia to taste

Dinner:
Mom's Vegetable Beef Soup

Toxicity Tip: For an effective deodorant mix 1/4 cup baking soda, 1/4 cup Arrowroot Powder, 5 Tbs. melted Coconut Oil and a few drops of any essential oils you choose. Pour into an old deodorant tube to cool and harden.

Max T3: Superfast Workout 4 – Surge

Day 19

Max Mind: Repeat this to yourself out any time you feel tempted to slip back to your old ways, especially if you are rationalizing or feeling sorry for yourself: "My commitment must be stronger than my emotions are at this moment." The pain of discipline is temporary but the pain of regret is permanent.

Eating Plan:

Breakfast:
Chocolate Power Smoothie

Snack:
Veggie Sticks with ranch dressing

Lunch:
Left over Mom's Vegetable Beef Soup

Snack:
Granny Smith apple with 1/2 cup Almond Butter

Dinner:
Jamie's Chicken Stir Fry

Max T3: Superfast Workout 5 – Upper Body

Day 20

Max Mind: One of our favorite quotes from Henry Ford: "If you think you can or think you can't, you're right." You CAN!

Eating Plan:

Breakfast:
Perfect French Vanilla Smoothie

Snack:
1/2 cup raw nuts and seeds

Lunch:
Chicken Breast Salad with 1/4 cup Olive Oil and 3 Tbs. Balsamic Vinegar

Snack:
Boiled Egg

Dinner:
South West Cod or Halibut
Mashed faux-potatoes
Green Salad

Toxicity Tip: If you are using butter to cook with, make sure it's organic so that you don't get any of the antibiotics or hormones used in dairy processing.

Max T3: Superfast Workout 6 – Lower Body

Day 21

Max Mind: Remember the old adage, "Failing to plan is planning to fail." It's a shopping an planning day. This is the most important step to making sure your week is a success.

Eating Plan:

Breakfast:
Scrambled Eggs with 2 slices turkey bacon

Snack:
1 cup Greek yogurt with 2 Tbs. chopped pistachios and 2 Tbs. Cacao nibs-Xylitol or Stevia to taste

Lunch:
Grilled Chicken Breast, black beans and salsa

Snack:
Granny Smith Apple with 1/4 cup Almond Butter

Dinner:
Tasty Teriyaki Salmon
Broccoli

Max T3: REST!

Day 22

Max Mind: Do something to celebrate your progress so far. If you've lost inches, go buy a new pair of pants that you couldn't have fit in before. Go climb the stairs that have always gotten you winded. Go for a hike that you couldn't do before. It feels good to see what all of your hard work has gotten you!

Eating Plan:

Breakfast:
Perfect French Vanilla Smoothie

Snack:
1/2 cup raw almonds

Lunch:
Chicken Breast Salad with 1/4 cup Olive Oil and 3 Tbs. Balsamic Vinegar

Snack:
3 to 5 celery sticks with 1/2 cup hummus

Dinner:
Classic Pot Roast with Sauerkraut

Max T3: Fast Workout 7 – Upper Body

Day 23

Max Mind: Your body is feeling amazing! Review your goals and see how close you are. The pain of discipline is far easier than the pain of regret. YOU can do this! Stay the course!

Eating Plan:

Breakfast:
Chocolate Power Smoothie

Snack:
Boiled Egg

Lunch:
Leftover Classic Pot Roast

Snack:
1/2 cup raw almonds

Dinner:
Juicy Grilled Steak with Bernaise sauce Sautéed Spinach, Kale, or Broccoli

Toxicity Tip: Read food labels and eliminate food additives and preservatives like MSG or aka's such as hydrolyzed vegetable protein, yeast extract, autolyzed yeast or sodium caseinate.

Max T3: Fast Workout 8 – Lower Body

Day 24

Max Mind: Pay it forward. Take your favorite thing that you've learned from this challenge and help someone else with it. Email a coworker a recipe. Show a family member how to cut down their exercise time. The best way to ensure your own success is to help someone else succeed.

Eating Plan:

Breakfast:
Berry Blast Smoothie

Snack:
3 to 5 celery sticks filled with Almond Butter

Lunch:
Chicken Breast Salad with 1/4 cup Olive Oil and 3 Tbs. Balsamic Vinegar

Snack:
1/2 cup walnuts

Dinner:
Black Bean Fiesta Soup

Max T3: Fast Workout 9 – Core

Day 25

Max Mind: Review your goals and see that you are almost at the finish line. Look at all the healthy habits you have created and the lifestyle changes you've made.

Eating Plan:

Breakfast:
Perfect French Vanilla Smoothie

Snack:
1/2 cup Pumpkin Seeds

Lunch:
Leftover Black Bean Fiesta Soup

Snack:
Boiled Egg

Dinner:
Jamie's Chicken Stir Fry

Toxicity Tip: The best body moisturizers are oils, like Jojoba, Almond or Coconut Oil.

Max T3: Fast Workout 10 – Surge

Day 26

Max Mind: If you aren't continually growing, you are dying. Find a book or website today that will give you more tools to continue in your new lifestyle. www.maximizedliving.com is a great place to start, so is your local bookstore.

Eating Plan:

Breakfast:
Unsweetend Greek yogurt and blueberries with 2 Tbs. Sliced almonds – Xylitol or Stevia to taste

Snack:
Veggie sticks with 1/2 cup hummus

Lunch:
Salmon Salad with 1/4 cup Olive Oil and 3 Tbs. Balsamic Vinegar

Snack:
Celery sticks with hummus

Dinner:
Vivian's Shepherd's Pie

Max T3: Fast Workout 11 – Upper Body

Day 27

Max Mind: Bill Cosby said, "I don't know the key to success, but the key to failure is trying to please everybody." Don't pay attention to people that are trying to pull you down. Surround yourself with people that lift you up! Who is it that you need to stop hanging out with?

Eating Plan:

Breakfast:
Chocolate Power Smoothie

Snack:
1/2 cup walnuts

Lunch:
Leftover Pellow's Shepherd's Pie

Snack:
Boiled Egg

Dinner:
Quick Baked Cod or Halibut
Mashed faux-potatoes
Green Salad

Max T3: Fast Workout 12 – Lower Body

Day 28

The NEW man or woman in the mirror: *What's your number now?*

Take the following test to find out how close you are to the cruise ship or nursing home. Take time to celebrate how far you've come and keep walking your new path!

	10 points	5 points	0 points
What's your BMI?	Less than 24	25-29	Over 30
What's your waist to hip ratio? (Waist is measured 1 in above navel, hips at widest point of buttocks)	.95 or below for men .80 or below for women	.96 to 1.0 for men .81 to .85 for women	1.0+ for men .85+ for women
How many medications are you taking?	0	1-2	More than 2
How many days a week do you skip breakfast?	0	1-2	More than 2
How many meals per week do you eat fast food?	0	1-2	More than 2
What is your resting pulse? (Beats per minute)	Less than 70	71-83	Over 83
How many times per week do you exercise?	More than 3	1-2	None
How many flu shots have you gotten?	Never	1-2	More than 2
How many sodas or sweetened beverages (tea, sports drinks, etc) do you drink per week?	0	1-2	More than 2
How many hours per night do you sleep?	8 or more	7	Less than 7

Where are you headed?
0-20 Sprinting towards the nursing home
21-40 It's time to get moving now
41-60 Assess your weak areas and get a plan
61-80 Stay consistent and keep improving
81-100 Keep it up and we'll see you on the cruise ship

Eating Plan:

Breakfast:
Berry Blast Smoothie

Snack:
Celery sticks with 1/2 cup hummus

Lunch:
Chinese cabbage salad with chicken

Snack:
1/2 cup raw almonds

Dinner:
Chicken Coconut Curry

Max T3: REST!

CHAPTER 10

Leave a Legacy

*"Nothing is more certain than the
victory of a man or a woman that never
quits or the failure of one that will."*

——*Author unknown*

Hope is what we want you to walk away with from this book—hope that you can turn your situation into triumph. The stories you read in this book were true stories of people who were just like you, or worse. If they could turn their bodies and their lives around, so can you!

Return the favor and inspire your friends and other people who read this book. If you feel like this book has changed your life, then we want to hear from you. Send your testimonial to **info@maximizedliving.com**.

Tens of thousands of ordinary people just like you are using this plan to transform their lives, so you are not alone. Go to **www.maximizedliving.com** to get help, get inspired, and to get involved.

It's time to really get started and apply what you know. Success is 20 percent knowledge and 80 percent change in behavior or action. As the great Martin Luther King Jr. said, "If you can't fly, run. If you can't run, walk. If you can't walk, crawl. But by all means keep moving!"

Testimonial — *Ed Rue, 29 years old*

Life Is Not About You

My life was changed forever on January 29, 2009. That was the day I checked myself into the emergency room on my way to a flight from Denver to Atlanta for my grandmother's funeral. Those plans were canceled when the doctor walked into the room and said, "Son, you have a blood clot. We need to hospitalize you immediately." This was probably the first time in my life I was really more than scared.

Here I am twenty-nine years old. My grandmother died. I can't go to the funeral. I was in the middle of a divorce. I was laid off from my job. I was home alone in an empty house with just me and my dog. On top of that, I was losing my home and now I'm sick. I thought that was bad, but then the really bad news came. The doctors came rushing in, hooked me up to oxygen, and said, "We looked at the X-rays and found that these clots have traveled to your lungs!" I was completely in shock. The next day they started me on two blood thinners, called Coumadin and Lovenox. That's when the real problems started.

Within two months of taking medication, I was diagnosed with high blood pressure. So now I was taking Coumadin and Metoprolol. This combination of drugs made me feel like I was having some sort of out of body experience. Every time I would take them I would pace around the house for hours at a time. I could not function properly, physically or mentally, while on these drugs. To make matters worse, they kept misdiagnosing me and giving more medication—Ativan, Topamax, Epidrin, Coumadin, Lovenox, Prilosec, Metoprolol, Hydrochlorothiazide, Neurontin, Amitriptyline, Hydrocodone, Sucralfate, nasal steroids, and there were more. I just don't want to bore you with the names.

By this time I was a little depressed and was crying often. The family members who were around me thought I was going crazy.

This was the point where I just knew I was dying slowly. I was in the emergency room so much that they sent me a letter that read: "Dear Edward Rue, you have visited the ER nine times within the past three weeks..." This was a letter stating that they thought I was going crazy because they couldn't figure out what was wrong with me.

By the grace of God, I was led to the Maximized Living Seminar. After the first hour of this seminar, I was blown away and was totally amazed. I was ready to start a new revolution.

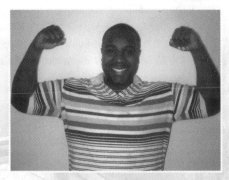

Since starting the program, I have lost over 50 pounds—and I'm off all medications. Let me say it again: I'm off all medications, eating healthy, exercising, and getting chiropractic adjustments. I have referred everyone I know, because I realize life is not about me but about serving others. I will continue to spread the news about Maximized Living until we change the world. My success that I have achieved is because I want to see others' success before my own success. Through my experience, I have dedicated my life to helping others see their true potential. I realize that by serving others, I am helping fulfill a bigger purpose of people reaching their God-given potential.

The Moral of the Story

"A person starts to live when he can live outside himself."[1]

—*Albert Einstein*

It's not about you. Two of the biggest selling books ever are the Bible and The Purpose Driven Life by Rick Warren. They both have one central message: it's not about you. Your life can't be about you or it will be empty. The worst chance you have of succeeding is making it about you. Did you know that 75 percent of what your children and those around you learn is not gained through your words but by your actions? You succeed best by expanding your vision to helping others. The acts of giving and kindness live at your core level. They make you human and give you a reason for your existence. Whether you fully realize it or not, you yearn every day to be a part of something bigger than yourself.

> People are counting on you to be successful and to help them transform their lives.

If you want to have your life mean something, it's important to understand that serving a greater purpose and living outside yourself is embedded in your DNA. You were quite literally born to make an imprint on the world. What's yours going to be?

Once you've succeeded at learning and applying the principles in this book, that success will affect the lives of thousands of people. People are counting on you to be successful and to help them transform their lives too.

Join the Mission

History has never been changed by the majority, but always by a small group of people committed to making a difference. The need for strong leaders to rise up and take charge of the health care in this country is now. Through the tools in this book, you can transform your family's and friends' lives. They, in turn, will influence their friends and families. If we get enough people believing in a vision of what health care should really be, together we'll influence and maybe even save millions around the world.

As you and the people around you get well, politicians will be forced to look at entire regions of the country where disease rates are at an all-time low. They'll want to know why so many are so well and health-care costs are so low. What they'll find are entire communities of people applying the Five Essentials to health and seeing the kind of results you read about in this book.

As you can see, together we can transform the health care of a country, all because you decided that you can do it. Most people think, "I can't make a difference," but you can.

Pass this book to someone you know and invite them to the next Maximized Living Makeover put on by your local Maximized Living doctor. Join the thousands of people currently transforming this country. Join the mission and help others who are desperately searching for answers, and join us as well. Nothing gives you a greater chance at personal success than helping others.

We are in this together, and we are more together than we are apart. You have the power to hand this book to somebody and change a life. Go to **www.maximizedliving.com** to find out more about joining the mission.

Grocery List Week 1 & 3

Produce:
Greens for salads
Garlic (1 head or chopped in a jar)
Bell Peppers-1 each red, yellow and green
Onions (3 per week)
Berries of your choosing, fresh or frozen
Broccoli (3 bunches)
Cauliflower (1 head)
Green onions   (1 bunch)
Soup vegetables-see list in recipe-can mix
   fresh and frozen
Granny Smith apples (2)
Mushrooms (1 container sliced)
Lime juice or 3 fresh limes
Pistachios (small container)
Pecans (1/4 cup)
Unsweetened coconut flakes (small
   container)
Celery (1 pack)
Almonds   (1 lb.)
Walnuts   (1/2 lb.)
Pumpkin and Sunflower Seeds (1 cup each)
Shallot (1)
Fresh Ginger (small section of fresh root, or
minced in a jar)

Meat, Poultry, Fish:
Ground beef or bison (2 to 4 lbs)
Chicken breasts (9 boneless, skinless)
Grass fed steak (1)
Turkey Bacon (no nitrates)
Cod or Halibut or other white fish (2 lbs.)
Salmon (2-1/4 lbs.)

Deli:
Hummus (1 container or make your own)

Dairy:
Greek yogurt (3 8 oz cartons)
Eggs (1 dozen)
Cheddar cheese (organic or raw, 8 oz.)
Coconut Milk

Canned Goods and Soup Aisle:
Tomatoes (chopped, 1 can)
Salsa (24 oz jar-look in Mexican section)
Black Beans (3 cans)
Water Chestnuts (1 small can) look in
   Asian section
Chicken Broth (1 carton, organic)
Tomato or Vegetable Juice (32 to 46 oz)

Condiments:
Bragg's Liquid Aminos (optional)
Grapeseed Vegenaise (1 jar)
Balsamic Vinegar
Tarragon Vinegar
Hot Sauce (check label for sugar and high
   fructose corn syrup)
Almond Butter
Salsa (at least 16 oz. jar)

Baking Aisle:
Almond Milk (1 carton) Use for mixing
   up scrambled eggs and can be used in
   mashed Fo-Tatoes
Vanilla Extract
Stevia or Xylitol (Stevia may be liquid or
   granular—liquid is very sweet so use
   sparingly)
Coconut Oil
Olive Oil (at least 16 oz.)

Miscellaneous:
Dry Sherry or you can use chicken broth
Cacao Nibs
Maximized Living Perfect Protein, Vanilla
and Chocolate

Spices:
Black Pepper
Oregano
Bay Leaves
Garlic Powder
Chili Powder
Cumin
Tarragon
Marjoram

Good salt-preferably Redman's Real Salt or another pink one. They have all the minerals left in them and do not cause the problems of sodium chloride. Do not use regular table salt!

These spices are all dried but feel free to use fresh ones if you wish. Use double the amount the recipe says if you do.

You probably have a lot of these spices and if you don't they will last a long time once you get them. Stock up on eggs, nuts and seeds, vegetable sticks (broccoli, bell peppers, celery) and almond butter as they make good snacks. Always keep chicken broth on hand to cook vegetables in-it improves the flavor. Adjust the amounts listed to fit the number of people you're cooking for and if you want leftovers. Most of these things can be found at regular grocery stores but for some you'll have to go the natural stores like Whole Foods, Sprouts, or SunFlower Market. Buy organic as much as possible and cage free eggs and grass fed beef. Stevia and Xylitol are the only allowed sugar substitutes. Stevia is used like Equal-a little goes a long way. Xylitol is used just like sugar and is better for baking.

Feel free to interchange the meals if you don't want something on a particular day. Always use breakfast as breakfast but the lunches and dinners are interchangeable. Most of the recipes freeze very well and make great lunches or dinners for later. If you don't like a particular dish you don't have to make it again. Use something else on the plan in its place. This is not a diet! It's the basis of an eating plan that will keep you healthy and trim to your 120th birthday!

Grocery List for Week 2

All of the staples from last week will not be repeated in this list. Oils, spices, etc. Check to see that you have enough.

Produce:
Greens for Salad (fills 1 gallon bag)
Cauliflower (2 heads)
Blueberries (fresh or frozen)
Sauerkraut (2 lb., check
  refrigerated section)
Kohlrabi or celeriac (celery root) 4 medium
Celery (1 pack)
Mushrooms (sliced, 3 packs)
Yellow Bell Pepper
Red Bell Pepper
Green Bell Pepper
Spinach (at least 2 lbs.)
Kale (1 bunch) optional
Broccoli (2-4 bunches)
Cilantro (1 bunch)
Berries (your choice, fresh or frozen)
Green Onions
Napa Cabbage (1 small)
Avocados (2)
Tomato (1)
Lime (1)
Vegetables for soup (see list in recipe and
  customize to your taste) You can use
  frozen.
Lemon Juice (or fresh lemons)
Ginger Root (fresh, small piece or minced
  in jar if you don't have any from last week)

Pecans
Raw Almonds (1 lb., whole, you can slice
  your own when called for)
Walnuts (1 cup)
Pumpkin Seeds (1 cup)

Meat, Poultry & Fish:
Chicken Breast (12 pcs boneless,skinless)
  Less if cooking for one or two
Rump Roast, Bottom Round, or Brisket
  (4 lb.) Less if cooking for one or two
Salmon (1 portion)
Steak (grass-fed, of your choice)
Beef or Bison (2 lbs.)
Cod or Halibut (or other white fish, 2 lb.)

Deli:
Hummus (16 oz. container) or make your
  own (Recipe in book. You just need 2
  cans chickpeas—you have everything
  else)

Dairy:
Real Butter
Greek Yogurt (1-1/2 cup)
Eggs (1 dozen)
Pint Cream or Milk (organic or raw)
Raw or organic cheddar cheese (8 oz.)

Canned Goods & Soup:
Soy or Tamari Sauce (also found with Asian
  food)
Dark Sesame Oil (also with Asian food)
Small can water chestnuts (check in Asian
  section)

Black Beans (3 cans)
Chicken or Beef Broth (4 cans or 2 cartons)
Chopped Tomatoes (1 can)

Condiments:

Baking Aisle:

Miscellaneous:
Large bottle of tomato or vegetable juice

20 in 30 Recipes

Salads

Chicken Salad – *Serves 4*

3-4 cups chopped cooked chicken
1 cup diced celery
2 Tbs. chopped green onions
1 Tbs. lemon juice
2/3 cup Vegenaise with Grapeseed Oil
1/4 cup walnuts or pecans, chopped
Salt and pepper

Mix all ingredients until combined and chill. Serve on lettuce or spinach leaves. To serve as a casserole, put in a lightly greased casserole, top with organic or raw parmesan or cheddar cheese and bake for 20 minutes 350 degrees.

Chinese Cabbage Salad

2 Tbs. soy sauce (tamari)
2 Tbs. Olive Oil
1 Tbs. fresh grated ginger
1 Small Napa cabbage cut into thin slices
1 Yellow bell pepper cut into thin strips
2 Tbs. dark Sesame Oil
2 Tbs. Sesame Seeds
3 cooked boneless skinless chicken breasts

In a small bowl, mix soy sauce, grated ginger, Sesame Oil and Olive Oil. Mix cabbage, bell pepper, add cooked chicken, drizzle with soy sauce mixture and sprinkle with Sesame Seeds.

Snacks

Guacamole – *Serves 4*

2 avocados
1 lime
2 clove garlic
1 small tomato
Salt, cumin and chili powder

Scoop out avocados into bowl and add lime juice, finely chopped garlic and chopped tomato. Mash it together and add spices to taste. Chill.

Hummus – *Serves 4*

2 cans rinsed chickpeas
3 cloves garlic
3 Tbs. Olive Oil
2 Tbs. lemon juice
Salt and cayenne pepper or paprika

Place all ingredients in food processor or blender until smooth. Taste and adjust seasoning.

Veggies

Sauteed Greens – Serves 2

1 Tbs. Coconut Oil
1/2 small onion
6 pitted black olives (optional)
2 lbs spinach, kale or collards (broccoli can be used if you parboil it first)
1 tsp lemon juice
3 cloves garlic (optional)
Salt and pepper
1/4 cup crumbled feta (optional)

Heat a large pan over medium high heat. Add oil and onion and cook til onion wilts. Add greens (you have to chop the kale or collards but not the spinach) and olives, if using them. Saute spinach 2-3 minutes and the rest of them 8-10 minutes. Add lemon juice, salt and pepper and cook one more minute. Sprinkle with feta if you like it.

Mashed No-tatoes – *Serves 4*

1 head cauliflower or several celery roots (celeriac)
1/4 cup butter
1/4 cup organic or raw half and half
Salt and pepper

Steam cauliflower in steamer or small amount of water until tender. Drain. In food processor, blend cauliflower or celery roots with remaining ingre-dients until smooth. You can't get this smooth enough without a blender or food processer. You'll be amazed how good this is!

Roasted Vegetables – *Serves 4*

Cut any vegetables you like-asparagus, Brussels sprouts, onions, green beans, tomatoes, broccoli, zucchini or yellow squash, or preferable all of these-into bite size pieces. Put in large roasting pan and toss with Olive Oil, chopped garlic and salt and pepper. Spread into thin layer and roast at 450 for about 30 minutes. You may want to turn them half way through. You'll wonder why you never liked veggies before! You can put a whole chicken in a roasting pan and roast for 1-1/2 hours and then sur-round it with veggies and roast for another 45 minutes. Double delicious and you have dinner all in one pan!

Soups

Black Fiesta Bean Soup – *Serves 4*

2 cans black beans
1 cup chicken stock
1/4 cup chopped onion
1/4 cup chopped green onions
3 cloves chopped garlic
2 tsp cilantro
2 Tbs. Coconut Oil
Salt, chili powder, cumin and hot sauce to taste.

In a food processor or blender puree 1 can black beans and the chicken stock. In a medium sauce pan sauté onions and garlic in oil. When veggies are tender add black bean mixture from blender, remaining can of black beans, and stir on medium low heat. Add spices a little at time and taste til you like it! Top with raw or organic cheddar.

Easy Advanced Plan Chili – *Serves 6*

1 Tbs. Coconut Oil
1/2 cup chopped onions
2 chopped garlic cloves
1-1/2 chopped celery
1 cup chopped green pepper
1-1/2 lbs ground beef or bison
2 tsp thyme leaves
2 tsp chili powder or more if you like
2 tsp cumin
Salt to taste
1 8oz can chopped tomatoes
1 12oz of salsa (all natural)

In large skillet, sauté onions, garlic, celery and pepper in oil til tender. Add meat, thyme, chili powder, and cumin and stir frequently for 5-6 minutes. Add salt, tomatoes and salsa to pot. Cover and simmer for an hour. This can also be cooked all day in the crockpot on low.

Mom's Vegetable Soup – *Serves 8 to 10*

Brown 1 to 2 lbs of ground beef or bison. Ad a whole chopped onion and 4 stalks of chopped celery and cook 5 minutes. Add salt and pepper to taste and 1 Tbs. marjoram. Add a 46 oz can of tomato juice and 2 cups chicken broth. Add whatever vegetables you like—broccoli, green baby lima beans, white beans, zucchini, yellow squash, okra, water chestnuts, mushrooms, any chopped greens, green beans, or cauliflower. Cook until tender-about 45 minutes. Adjust seasonings to taste.

Sauces, Salad Dressings and Smoothies

Hollandaise Sauce

Put 3 eggs in blender on low. Add 1/2 cup melted butter, 2 Tbs. lemon juice, 1/4 tsp salt and a pinch of cayenne. Blend until smooth and thickened, about 20 seconds. To make Bernaise sauce, just add 1 Tbs. Tarragon Vinegar, 1 tsp tarragon, 1 tsp shallots or onion, and pepper.

Berry Blast Smoothie – *Serves 1*

The basic smoothie is 1 scoop whey protein powder, 1 cup Coconut Milk, and Stevia to taste if your protein isn't sweetened.   2 raw eggs can be used instead of the protein powder.
Add 1 cup frozen berries
If your fruit isn't frozen just add some ice cubes. Blend and enjoy!

Chocolate Power Smoothie – *Serves 1*

3/4 scoop chocolate whey protein powder
1 cup unsweetened coconut or Almond Milk
1 cup ice
Stevia or Xylitol to taste
(You can also add 1 Tbs. of almond butter)

Perfect French Vanilla Smoothie – *Serves 1*

3/4 scoop protein powder or 2 whole raw eggs
1/2 can unsweetened, full fat Coconut Milk
1 cup ice
2 capfuls vanilla extract
Stevia or Xylitol to taste

Put it all in blender and blend until frothy.

Main Dishes

Classic Pot Roast with Sauerkraut – *Serves 6*

4 lb rump roast, bottom round or brisket
Salt and pepper
2 Tbs. Coconut Oil
3/4 cup chopped onions
1 tsp thyme leaves
1/4 tsp oregano
2 lb sauerkraut
2 bay leaves
2 cups beef or chicken broth
4 med kohlrabi or celery roots, peeled and quartered
2 cups chopped tomatoes or 1 can diced
4 stalks celery

Season the beef with salt and pepper. In a large Dutch oven, melt Coconut Oil and brown meat with the onions. Add thyme. Cover with sauerkraut, tomatoes, and bay leaves. Simmer several hours til tender. Add veggies after about 1-1/2 hours. Cover and continue to simmer. This can be made in a crockpot after you brown the meat.

Coconut Curry Chicken – *Serves 4*

2 lbs boneless skinless chicken breast
1 can Coconut Milk
2 cups broccoli
1 cup mushrooms
1 onion
1 Tbs. curry powder
1 tsp minced garlic
1 tsp minced ginger
Salt to taste

In a large skillet. Add Coconut Milk, chicken, broccoli. Mushrooms, and chopped onion. Cook on medium high 15 minutes. Add curry powder, garlic, ginger and salt cook over medium low heat for 15 minutes. Garnish with fresh parsley.

Jamie's Chicken Stir Fry – *Serves 4 to 6*

2 lbs boneless skinless chicken breast cut into cubes
1 small can water chestnuts
2 cups broccoli
1 cup sliced red bell peppers
3/4 cup sliced onions
1 cup sliced mushrooms
2 Tbs. Coconut Oil
1 tsp salt

In a large wok or skillet, heat oil. Add chicken and cook on medium heat for 5 minutes. Add broccoli, peppers, onions, mushrooms, and salt. Cook until veggies are crisp tender and chicken is done. Can be topped with tamari sauce or Bragg's liquid aminos.

Baked Cod or Halibut – *Serves 4*
2 lbs Cod or Halibut
Juice of 1 lemon
2 Tbs. butter
1 tsp salt
1 tsp parsley flakes
1 tsp garlic powder
Coconut Oil

Coat bottom of baking dish with oil and put in Cod or Halibut. Pour lemon juice over fish. Top with butter, parsley, salt and garlic powder. Bake at 400 about 15 minutes or until the fish easily flakes.

Southwestern Cod or Halibut – *Serves 4*

2 lbs Cod or Halibut
4 Tbs. lime juice
1 cup salsa
1 tsp salt
Coconut Oil

Place Cod or Halibut in oiled baking pan and sprinkle with lime juice and salt. Top with salsa. Bake at 400 until fish flakes, about 20 minutes.

Tasty Teriyaki Salmon – *Serves 4*
For sauce:
1/4 cup tamari sauce
1/4 cup dry sherry
1 Tbs. Sesame Oil
1 Tbs. grated ginger root
2 minced cloves garlic

For fish:
2 lbs salmon-wild caught is best

Lemon wedges

Combine sauce ingredients. Place fish is glass dish and pour the sauce on. Marinate in the fridge for 2 hours. Grill the fish or broil in oven. Cook 3-4 minutes each side while basting with sauce. Serve fish with lemon wedges.

Vivian's Shepherd's Pie – *Serves 4 to 6*
2 lbs ground beef or bison
1/2 cup chopped onion
1/2 cup chopped celery
1/2 cup chopped bell pepper
1 cup mushrooms, sliced
Any veggies you have on hand
Salt and pepper to taste
Any herbs you like-marjoram, thyme, Season All, etc.

Brown beef or bison with onion and celery. Add mushrooms and cook for 5 minutes. Add the other veggies, (chopped greens, broccoli, chopped snow peas, zucchini, squash, green peas in any combination). Cook for a few minutes and add a little beef or chicken broth. Thicken with some arrowroot. Put in a 9x13 baking dish and top with mashed faux-tatoes. Bake for 30 minutes at 350 and dig in!

Optional Treats

Taco Salad – *Serves 4*

1 lb ground beef or bison
1/2 cup chopped onion
1/2 cup chopped red pepper
1/2 cup chopped mushrooms
1 tsp salt
1 tsp Bragg's Liquid Aminos
1 tsp chili powder
Spinach leaves
Bean Sprouts
1 can black beans
1 large chopped tomato
1 red bell pepper cut in strips
1/2 cup pitted olives
Guacamole or salsa

Mix meat, onion, chopped pepper, mushrooms, salt, Bragg's and chili powder together. You can either form into patties and grill them or sauté it all together. To make the salad, place a handful of spinach on a plate, top with bean sprouts, black beans, tomato, strips of pepper, and olives. Place grilled burger or sautéed meat on top. You can add hot sauce if desired. Eat with guacamole or salsa.

Salad Dressing

Combine Olive Oil with Balsamic Vinegar, salt and pepper for the base. You can add some Dijon mustard or any herbs you like. Olive Oil and lemon juice is a nice light dressing. Olive Oil and Red Wine Vinegar with oregano is a classic. Olive Oil, lemon juice and an avocado is a good substitute for Green Goddess dressing.

Cheese Drop Biscuits

4 eggs
1/4 cup Coconut Oil
1/4 tsp salt
1/4 tsp onion powder
1/3 cup sifted Coconut Flour
1/4 tsp baking powder
1/4 cup parmesan cheese
1/3 cup shredded sharp cheddar
Garlic and herb seasoning

Blend eggs, oil, salt and onion powder. Combine Coconut Flour with baking powder and whisk. Combine with wet ingredients and fold in cheese. Drop batter by tablespoons onto greased cookie sheet. Sprinkle with garlic and herb seasoning. Bake at 400 degrees for 12 to 14 minutes.

Blueberry Pancakes – *Serves 2*

2 scoops vanilla protein powder
2 Tbs. whole ground Flaxseed meal
6 Tbs. Coconut Flour
1/4 tsp baking powder
1/4 tsp salt
1/2 tsp Stevia
4 eggs
1 cup milk
4 Tbs. butter
1 pint blueberries
Generous sprinkling of cinnamon
Grapeseed Oil spray

Mix ingredients together except blueberries. Spray preheated pan with oil. Drop batter on hot pan. Drop blueberries throughout. Flip over when they are set. Butter and eat plain or top with blueberry syrup by cooking some blueberries with a little water and Stevia. You can make the topping with any kind of berries.

Coconut Macaroons

1 cup raw almonds
2 cups raw unsweetened flaked coconut
1/4 cup protein powder
2 to 3 Tbs. unsweetened cocoa powder
Stevia or Xylitol to taste
6 to 9 Tbs. warmed liquid Coconut Oil
2 Tbs. Flaxseeds

In blender or food processor, grind almonds and Flaxseeds. Blend in remaining ingredients. Remove mixture and place tablespoon sized serving on cookie sheet and chill. Makes 12.

Zucchini Casserole – *Serves 6*

2 small zucchini
2 lbs ground meat
1/2 onion, chopped
3 cloves garlic, chopped
3 eggs
2 Tbs. Bragg's liquid aminos
2 15 oz cans tomato sauce
2 7 oz cans tomato paste
1 pint ricotta cheese
Pinch of Stevia
Salt and pepper to taste

Mix in glass bowl, Bragg's, garlic, onion, 2 eggs and ground meat. Flatten mixture into 9 by 4 inch glass casserole dish. Slice zucchini and lay over meat. Mix ricotta, one egg, salt and pepper and spread over zucchini. Mix tomato paste and sauce with Stevia and pour over ricotta. Bake 1-1/2 hours at 350 degrees.

CHAPTER 11

NOTES

Introduction

What This Book Is and What This Program Can Do for You

1. Raold Dahl, Willy Wonka and the Chocolate Factory, DVD, directed by Mel Stuart (1971; n.p.: Warner Home Video, 1997).

Chapter 1

Cruise Ship or Nursing Home?—Your Road Map to a Maximized Life

1. Ron Osborn, Jeff Reno, Kevin Wade, and Bo Goldman, Meet Joe Black, directed by Martin Brest (1998; n.p.: Universal Pictures).

Chapter 2

You've Been Lied To!

1. "Truth," TwainQuotes.com, http://www.twainquotes.com/Truth.html (accessed December 21, 2009).

2. Associated Press, "Medical Bills Make Up Half of Bankruptcies" MSNBC.com, http://www.msnbc.msn.com/id/6895896/ (accessed December 21, 2009).

3. Ibid.

Chapter 3

Step One Toward the Cruise Ship—A Maximized Mind Is Your Secret Weapon

1. "Quotation #407 from Michael Moncur's (Cynical) Quotations," QuotationsPage.com, http://www.quotationspage.com/quote/407.html (accessed December 21, 2009).

2. "Cancer Statistics and Views of Causes," Science News 115, no. 2 (January 13, 1979): 23, http://www.jstor.org/pss/3963979 (accessed December 21, 2009).

3. Bruce Lipton, PhD, Biology of Belief (n.p., Hay House, 2008).

4. Bradley J. Willcox, MD, D. Craig Willcox, PhD, and Makoto Suzuki, MD, The Okinawa Diet Plan (n.p., Three Rivers Press, 2005).

Chapter 4

Why You Can't Lose Weight—What You Don't Know Will Hurt You, or at Least Keep You Fat

1. University of California Agriculture and Natural and Resources, "Nutrition Online Media Kit," http://news .ucanr.org/mediakits/Nutrition/nutritionfactsheet.shtml (accessed December 24, 2009).

2. Ron Rosedale, MD, "Burn Fat, Not Sugar to Lose Weight" http://www.drrosedale.com/resources/pdf/Burn%20Fat,%20Not%20Sugar%20to%20lose%20weight.pdf (accessed December 21, 2009).

3. Dr. Richard E. Tapert, "Stop Worrying About Cholesterol: Book Excerpt," AvoidHeartAttack.com, http://www.avoidheartattack.com/755280.html (accessed December 21, 2009); findings summarized from K. M. Anderson, W. P. Castelli, D. Levy, " Cholesterol and Mortality," Journal of the American Medical Association 257, no. 16 (April 24, 1987): 2176–2180.

4. Ibid.

5. Sally Fallon and Mary G. Enig, PhD, "Diet and Disease: Not What You Think," http://www.coconut-info.com/diet_and_disease.htm (accessed December 21, 2009).

6. "Side Effects," Crestor.com, http://www.crestor.com/c/explore-crestor/side-effects.aspx (accessed December 21, 2009).

7. "Quotation #487 from Michael Moncur's (Cynical) Quotations," QuotationsPage.com, http://www.quotationspage.com/quote/487.html (accessed December 21, 2009).

8. Dwight Lundell, "Twenty-Five-Year Heart Surgeon Reveals the Statin Scam," Wellsphere, April 9, 2009, http://stanford.wellsphere.com/healthy-living-article/25-year-heart-surgeon-reveals-the-statin-scam/640314 (accessed December 21, 2009).

9. Ibid.

10. Ibid.

Chapter 5

Step Two Toward the Cruise Ship—Lose Ten Pounds Fast

1. "Famous Quotes from Frank, Annlies Mary," S9.com: Biographical Dictionary, http://www.s9.com/Biography/Frank-Annlies-Mary (accessed December 21, 2009).

2. Tom Tai-Seale and Coleman Chandler, "Nutrition and Overweight Concerns in Rural Areas," http://www .srph.tamhsc.edu/centers/rhp2010/09Volume1nutrition.pdf (accessed December 21, 2009).

3. Janice Kaszursky, "People Still Getting Fatter—Over One Billion Adults Overweight Worldwide," http://ezinearticles.com/?People-Still-Getting-Fatter---Over-1-Billion-Adults-Overweight-Worldwide&id=306686 (accessed December 21, 2009).

4. Ibid.

5. Ben Lerner, Greg Loman, and Charles Majors, Maximum Living Makeover (Orlando, FL: Maximized Living Publishing, 2008), 60.

6. Ibid.

Chapter 6
Step Three Toward the Cruise Ship—Turn Your Power On!

1. Daniel J. DeNoon, "Chiropractic Cuts Blood Pressure," WedMD Health News, March 16, 2007, http://www.webmd.com/hypertension-high-blood-pressure/news/20070316/chiropractic-cuts-blood-pressure (accessed December 21, 2009).

2. G. Bakris, M. Dickholtz, P. M. Meyer, et al, "Atlas Vertebrae Realignment and Achievement of Arterial Pressure Goal in Hypertensive Patients: a Pilot Study," Journal of Human Hypertension 21 (March 2007): 347–352.

3. G. Bakris, M. Dickholtz, P. M. Meyer, et al, "Atlas Vertebrae Realignment and Achievement of Arterial Pressure Goal in Hypertensive Patients: a Pilot Study," Journal of Human Hypertension 21 (March 2007): 347–352.

4. H. Winsor, "Sympathetic Segmental Disturbances-11: The Evidence of the Association in Dissected Cadaver of Visceral Disease with Vertebral Deformities of the Same Sympathetic Segments," Medical Times 49 (November 1921): 267–271.

5. Kentaro Shimizu, MD, "Spinal Kyphosis Causes Demyelination and Neuronal Loss in the Spinal Cord," Spine Journal 30, no. 21 (November 1, 2005): 2388–2392.

6. Deborah M. Kado, MD, Arun S. Karlamangla, MD, Elizabeth Barrett-Connor, MD and Gail A. Greendale, MD, "Hyperkyphotic Posture Predicts Mortality in Older Community-Dwelling Men and Women: A Prospective Study," Journal of the American Geriatrics Society 52, no. 10 (October 2004): 1662; Shimizu, Kentaro MD, "Spinal Kyphosis Causes Demyelination and Neuronal Loss in the Spinal Cord," Spine Journal 30, no. 21 (November 1, 2005): 2388–2392.

7. C. A. Lantz, "The Subluxation Complex," Foundations of Chiropractic: Subluxation, Meridel Gatterman, ed. (n.p.: Mosby Year Book, 1995); C. A. Lance, "Immobilization Degeneration and the Fixation Hypotheses of the Chiropractic Subluxation," Chiropractic Research Journal 1, no. 1 (1998).

8. Haymo W. Thiel, DC, PhD; Jennifer E. Bolton, E. PhD; Sharon Docherty, PhD, and Jane C. Portlock, PhD, "Safety of Chiropractic Manipulation of the Cervical Spine: A Prospective National Survey," Spine Journal 32, no. 21 (October 1, 2007): 2375–2378.

9. "Tony Robbins Quotes," BrainyQuote.com, http://www.brainyquote.com/quotes/quotes/t/tonyrobbin173238.html (accessed December 21, 2009).

Chapter 7
Step Four Toward the Cruise Ship—Stop Poisoning Your Family!

1. "Tom Krause Quotes," ThinkExist.com, http://thinkexist.com/quotation/if-you-don-t-want-it-bad-enough-to-risk-losing-it/763349.html (accessed December 21, 2009).

2. California Department of Developmental Services, "2003 DDS Autism Report," http://www.dds.ca.gov/autism (accessed December 24, 2009).

3. Centers for Disease Control, Autism and Developmental Disabilities Monitoring Network, "Morbidity and Mortality Weekly Report: Prevalence of Autism Spectrum Disorders," February 9, 2007, http://www.cdc .gov/MMWR/preview/mmwrhtml/ss5601a2.htm (accessed December 24, 2009).

4. Centers for Disease Control, "Autism Spectrum Disorders: Data and Statistics," http://www.cdc.gov/ncbddd/autism/data.html (accessed December 24, 2009).

5. "Pharma's New Enemy: Clean Living," Forbes, November 29, 2004.

6. Ibid.

7. Ibid.

8. Joseph Mercola, "Using Aspirin and Ibuprofen Can Increase Your Breast Cancer Risk by 50 Percent," June 16, 2005, http://articles.mercola.com/sites/articles/archive/2005/06/16/pain-killers.aspx (accessed December 21, 2009); as quoted in Journal of the National Cancer Institute 97, no. 11 (June 1, 2005): 805–812.

9. "Medicines to Reduce Breast Cancer Risk: Tamoxifen," American Cancer Society, http://www.cancer.org/docroot/cri/content/cri_2_6x_tamoxifen_and_raloxifene_questions_and_answers_5.asp (accessed December 21, 2009).

10. Dan Childs and Raja Jagadeesan, MD, "Doctors Applaud Infant Cold/Cough Drug Recall," ABC News Medical Unit, October 11, 2007, http://abcnews.go.com/Health/Drugs/story?id=3718265&page=2 (accessed December 21, 2009).

11. Organic Consumer Association, "How Toxic Are Your Household Cleaning Supplies?" http://www.organicconsumers.org/articles/article_279.cfm (accessed December 24, 2009).

12. Hardick Chiropractic Services, Patient Resources, http://www.hardickchiropractic.com/Personal CareProducts.pdf (accessed December 21, 2009); adapted from NTP. Seventh Annual Report on Carcinogens. U.S. Department of Health and Human Services, Public Health Service, National Institute of Environmental Health Sciences, Technical Resources, inc. Rockville, MD, 1994.

13. "Material Safety Data Sheet: Propylene glycol MSDS," ScienceLab.com, http://www.sciencelab.com/xMSDS-Propylene_glycol-9927239 (accessed December 24, 2009).

14. Journal of the American College of Toxicology 2, no. 7 (1983), reprinted by Healthy-Communications.com, http://www.healthy-communications.com/journal_of_the_american_college_.html (accessed December 28, 2009).

15. Joseph Mercola, "Teflon Chemicals Are a Threat to Health," Mercola.com, August 25, 2004, http://article .mercola.com/sites/articles/archive/2004/08/25/teflon-chemicals.aspx (accessed December 24, 2009).

16. International Journal of Cancer 18, no. 8 (April 15, 2006): 2040–2047.

17. Jasmine Jafferali, "Harmful Ingredients Found in Bottled Water," Chicago Family Health Examiner, July 12, 2009, http://www.examiner.com/x-7158-Chicago-Family-Health-Examiner~y2009m7d12-Is-your-bottled-water-safe (accessed December 12, 2009).

18. "The Bottled Water Myth," EcoPlasticBottles.com, http://ecoplasticbottles.com/a328031-the-bottled-water-myth.cfm (accessed December 28, 2009).

19. "Patients: FAQs," International Academy of Oral Medicine and Toxicology (IAOMT) http://www.iaomt.org/patients/index.asp (accessed December 24, 2009).